ITALIAN MEDITERRANEAN DIET FROM APPETIZERS TO DESSERTS FOR BEGINNERS

The Last Complete Recipe Book Of The Italian Mediterranean Diet, The Tastiest Recipes To Lose Weight, In An Easy, Fast And Without Too Many Sacrifices. Eating Well To Feel In Shape.

Alberto Garofano

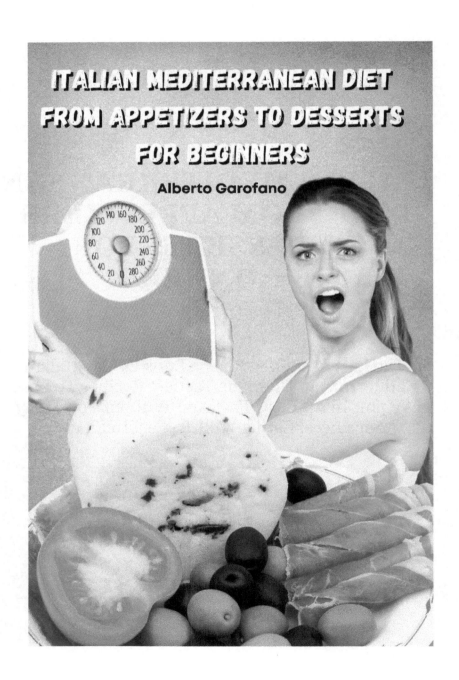

Table Of Contents

INTRODUCTION

With southern European delicacies to your desired weight: This is what the Mediterranean diet promises. We say whether it works, what exactly this diet is and what should be looked for. Because who doesn't want to indulge in culinary delights and bring the holiday home to their plate. Right, everyone probably would.
What is actually behind the Mediterranean diet, which foods are allowed and which advantages and disadvantages the diet brings with it, we explain to you here. Fried fish and vegetables with a view of the sea - most people probably find the thought of it a dream. Eating like you're on vacation sounds promising, doesn't it? The Mediterranean diet is based on exactly this principle and looks our southern European neighbors on the plate. Find out what is behind the Mediterranean diet, how and if it works here.
What is the Mediterranean Diet?
A balanced, healthy, varied and tasty diet is the basis of the Mediterranean diet. Here, the habits of the Mediterranean are adopted. Strictly speaking, however, the Mediterranean diet is not a real diet, but rather a form of nutrition and lifestyle in which fiber-rich mixed foods and fresh ingredients are on the menu. In addition, care is taken to ensure that the individual meals are eaten slowly and comfortably. A slow weight loss of two kilograms per month is promised. The concept is more of a healthy diet than a diet. To lose weight, you should count calories and use olive oil sparingly.

The Mediterranean diet mainly features high-fiber and fresh ingredients on the menu - based on our neighbors from the south.
How does the Mediterranean diet work?
A fiber-rich mixed diet with healthy fats and lots of fresh ingredients such as vegetables, Mediterranean salads, fish and fresh fruit should make our body slim. The Mediterranean diet scores with many valuable ingredients that regulate blood lipids and reduce the risk of cardiovascular diseases. Vegetables, fruits and salads are good for digestion. But pasta, bread, rice, legumes and cold-pressed olive oil, fresh herbs and garlic are also on the menu.
Important in the Mediterranean diet program: to take time to eat. A slow and relaxed meal is therefore very important. The southern Europeans take a lot of time, always cook and eat with great pleasure. A clever strategy - studies have now also proven this: Eating slowly helps you lose weight. Because if you don't take your time, you often miss the body's natural feeling of satiety and consume unnecessary calories. In addition, Mediterranean food ensures a balanced fat metabolism and, according to studies, lowers the cholesterol level . In addition, scientific research shows a positive correlation between the Mediterranean diet and the prevention of Alzheimer's disease. A study from the USA was able to show that foods such as vegetables, fruit, olive oil and the like can lower the risk of Alzheimer's disease.

The Mediterranean diet does not provide for an additional sports program. Counting calories is also not the order of the day - you can eat your fill with the right foods. Ideally, these should always be freshly prepared.

The fresh ingredients in the Mediterranean diet can reduce the risk of cardiovascular disease. By eating slowly and relaxed, the feeling of satiety can be better perceived and unnecessary calories can be saved.

It Is Better To Avoid These Foods

This includes only two food groups:

- red meat and its products (often very fatty and therefore unsuitable)
- fatty dairy products such as double cream cheese and cream cheese

You Can Consume These Foods

The main components of the Mediterranean diet are mainly ingredients that are regularly consumed in the Mediterranean region. This includes:

- fresh salads and lots of vegetables
- Fresh fish and / or seafood several times a week
- fruit
- good, cold-pressed olive oil
- plenty of fresh herbs and garlic
- poultry
- Rice and pasta
- Legumes such as chickpeas or lentils (slow rise in blood sugar levels)
- Almonds

- Low-fat dairy products such as goat and sheep milk or products (high calcium content, have anti-inflammatory effects)
- Wholemeal bread, wholemeal flatbread, sourdough bread (makes the blood sugar rise only slowly and thus makes you feel full for longer)
- Red wine in moderation (anti-aging effect due to the numerous antioxidants present)

This is the right way to get started
To change the previous diet to a Mediterranean diet, it is initially easier if you follow a few tips. We have put together the most important ones for you:
- Season the meals with herbs instead of salt: A high consumption of salt carries the risk of cardiovascular diseases.
- Nuts as a snack for in between: fill you up for a long time and provide valuable fats.
- Poultry instead of red meat: If you don't want to do without meat, you can simply buy a portion of poultry instead of red meat. This also provides a lot of proteins .
- Use sheep and goat's milk products instead of high-fat cow's milk products: These are much lower in fat.
- Allow a lot of time for the preparation and consumption of meals (the more time you take to eat, the less food you eat. Because eating too quickly, you consume significantly more food until you feel full)

With a few simple tips and tricks such as herbs instead of salt or almonds for cravings, the Mediterranean diet can be wonderfully integrated into your everyday diet.

The Benefits Of The Mediterranean Diet
Many people think that the Mediterranean diet is one of the healthiest nutritional concepts. The large amount of fruit and vegetables generates a high intake of vitamins and minerals and is therefore very balanced and varied. In combination with exercise, the Mediterranean diet is very suitable for a long-term change in diet and healthy weight loss.
The ingredients of the Mediterranean diet are also available in every supermarket in winter. Eating out is also absolutely no problem due to the variety of "permitted" foods.
The Cons Of The Mediterranean Diet
The concept of the Mediterranean Diet is more of a healthy diet than a diet. An integrated sports program is not intended for this. Nevertheless, a slow weight loss of two kilograms per month is promised. However, this can only be guaranteed in combination with sport.

You should also count calories and pay attention to the amount of olive oil used in order to generate actual weight loss. Breakfast should not be taken over by the habits of our southern neighbors. Often only a cup of coffee is drunk and pastries are consumed, which in turn leads to a rapid rise in blood sugar levels. A short time later, hunger can return. As an alternative, muesli and / or yogurt and fresh fruit are suitable. In addition, the Mediterranean seafood diet is not very cheap and takes a lot of time to prepare meals, which is another disadvantage.

The Mediterranean diet is considered by many experts to be one of the healthiest diets, as it provides us with the best possible supply through a high intake of vitamins and minerals. However, the diet does not provide for an integrated sports program.

For Whom Is The Mediterranean Diet Suitable

Suitable for:

- All connoisseurs who primarily strive for a healthy and balanced diet, with weight loss as the highest priority
- The Mediterranean diet is suitable for all ages and target groups

Smart Tips

If you keep an eye on the calories and eat a Mediterranean salad more often, for example, you can eat quite healthily with the Mediterranean diet. If you also exercise, you can lose weight in a healthy way. The regularity is crucial here. At best, make exercise an integral part of your life.

Even if you are healthy, from a diet point of view you should use some ingredients of the Mediterranean diet sparingly, for example the high-calorie olive oil. Although this offers high-quality ingredients, if consumed in larger quantities can lead to weight gain.

In addition, it can be helpful to plan meals carefully in order to keep an eye on the calories as described above. It is best to choose varied dishes within a week. This not only gives you various important vitamins and minerals, but also brings variety to your plate.

⭐ *55% OFF for BookStore NOW at $ 30,95 instead of $ 41,95!* ⭐

The Italian Mediterranean Diet cuisine is one of

the best cuisines in the world in this cookbook I

propose the most delicious recipes for both

appetizers and desserts, spoil your palate and

increase your culinary skills.

Buy is NOW and let your Customers get addicted

to this amazing book!

Buy is NOW and let your Customers get addicted to this amazing book!

START

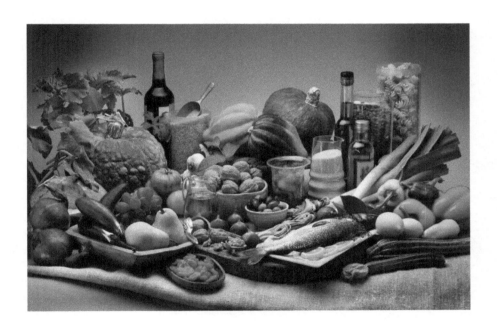

OLIVE ALL'ASCOLANA OR STUFFED FRIED OLIVES

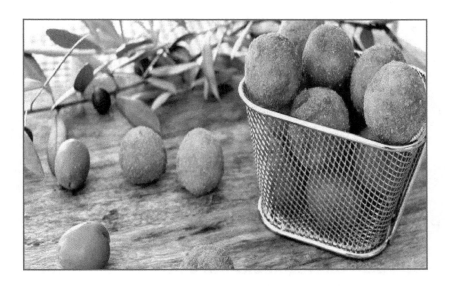

Serving: 4

INGREDIENTS

- For the filling
- 75 g Minced beef
- 75 g Minced pork
- 1 small of Onion
- 1 small carrot
- Celery (I haven't put it)
- Extra virgin olive oil 30 g
- White wine half a glass
- Egg 1
- 40 g Sliced bread or bread crumbs

- 40 g Grated Parmesan cheese
- Peel of half a lemon
- Salt
- Nutmeg
- Pepper
- To batter and fry
- Flour
- 3 Eggs
- Bread crumbs
- Oil half a liter
-

PREPARATION

1. Chop the vegetables. In a little oil, sauté the onion over medium heat first and when it is golden add the carrot. Let cook for a few minutes.
2. Add the minced meats and cook for a few minutes over moderate heat, when it is golden add white wine and let it evaporate. Add salt, pepper and nutmeg and cook for another couple of minutes. Remove from the fire and let it warm.
3. While you rinse the olives so that they lose excess salt, remove the bones if necessary.
4. When the sauce is warm, put it in a mincer or in a robot with all the other ingredients and grind it until the mixture is fine and homogeneous. Lemon peel is better if you add it already grated. It should be a soft dough, but if you see

that it has been left with some liquid and sticky you can add a little grated

5. Parmesan or breadcrumbs.
6. Take an olive and fill it as much as you can with the dough you have prepared. You can help yourself with a butter knife and a finger.
7. Coat the olives with flour, egg and bread. And again just for egg and bread so that they are left with an even layer.
8. When you pass them on the bread the second time, mold the olive in your palms as if it were a meatball so that they take a round shape.
9. Fry the olives in plenty of oil until golden brown, drain on absorbent paper and ready to serve.

Italian meatballs

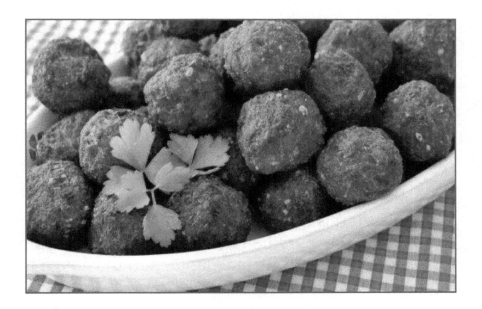

Servings 4

INGREDIENTS

- Minced beef (or 50% beef and 50% pork) 500 g
- Stale bread soaked 1/3 of a bar or a medium cooked potato (for celiacs)
- Grana padano or parmiggiano or grated old sheep cheese 70 g
- Eggs 2
- Salt
- Pepper
- Oregano
- Parsley some leaves

- Garlic 1 small clove
- Wine (optional)
- Milk (optional)
- Olive oil go for frying

PREPARATION

1. Soak the bread with milk or water. When it is very soft, squeeze it well so that it releases all the liquid. Celiacs can use gluten-free bread or a medium cooked potato passed through a pureed raisin.
2. Put all the ingredients in a bowl and mix until everything is well amalgamated. If the dough is hard, add a little wine, milk or water. If it's sticky add a little breadcrumbs. Let stand 10 minutes.
3. Begin to form walnut-sized meatballs.
4. Heat the oil and when it is very hot add the Italian meatloaf, 6-8 units a few at a time, so that the temperature of the oil does not drop too much and so that they come out crispy. Do not stir. It is ideal that the meatballs are almost covered by the oil. Fry for a couple of minutes, then flip it over and fry for another minute.
5. Drain them on a steel colander or on paper, then transfer to a plate. They are ready for you to enjoy.

Artichokes with the perfume of good grass

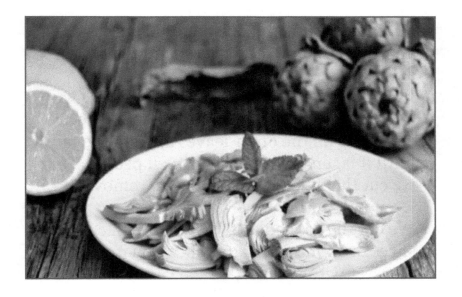

Servings 4

INGREDIENTS

- 8 Artichokes
- 2 glasses Vinegar
- 1 L Water
- Salt
- Good grass
- Extra virgin olive oil

PREPARATION

1. Put in a bowl plenty of water and a glass of vinegar or lemon, here we will add the artichokes as we clean them.
2. In a saucepan put a liter of water to boil.
3. While we are cleaning the artichokes. We are removing all the outer leaves and cut the tail until it is tender and leave it well peeled. Then we cut the tip of the artichoke to remove the less tender part of the leaves.
4. We cut the artichoke in half and then cut it into slices of about 3 mm and put them in our bowl of water with vinegar.
5. As soon as the water boils, add a glass of vinegar.
6. We wait for it to boil again and then we put the artichokes well drained.
7. We wait for the water to start boiling again and we count 30 seconds.
8. We drain and let cool.
9. When they are very cold, we season them with salt and oil, mix well and decorate with a little good grass.

Sweet and sour aubergines with raisins and pine nuts

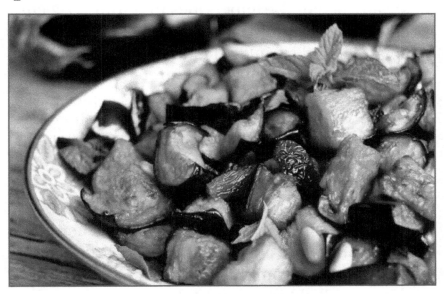

Servings 4

INGREDIENTS

- 500 g Black aubergines
- Salt
- 20 g Pine nuts
- 20 g Raisins
- Garlic 1 clove
- Apple cider vinegar 50 ml (or white wine vinegar for a more intense flavor)
- Sugar 5 g / (half a teaspoon)
- Olive oil see
- Mint leaves

PREPARATION

1. Wash and cut the aubergines first into 1.5-2 cm slices and then into cubes. Put them in a colander and sprinkle them evenly with coarse salt. Let stand 1 hour (minimum 30 minutes).
2. Rinse the aubergines under the tap, squeeze them well with your hands to drain all the liquid, and then dry them with paper or a clean kitchen towel.
3. Soak the raisins in a little water for about 20 minutes.
4. Put plenty of oil in a wide frying pan, when it is very hot, fry the aubergines little by little, stirring them from time to time so that they are done on all sides and until they are golden brown. Drain them on absorbent paper and reserve.
5. When you have all the aubergines ready, toast the pine nuts in a clean pan and set them aside.
6. Crush an unpeeled garlic clove with a knife and put it in the pan with a thread of oil, heat over medium-low heat for about 3 minutes so that the oil takes on flavor, then remove the garlic.
7. Put the aubergines in the pan and sauté a little. Add the toasted pine nuts and the well drained re-hydrated raisins.
8. In a glass dissolve the sugar with the vinegar, add it to the aubergines and cook until the liquid has completely evaporated. Adjust the salt, add some mint leaves and stir (this mind

will turn black but it gives it a lot of flavor, then you can remove it and add fresh mint).

9. Serve the sweet and sour aubergines with cold raisins and pine nuts. You can decorate the plate with some fresh mint leaves.

Cheese bonbons

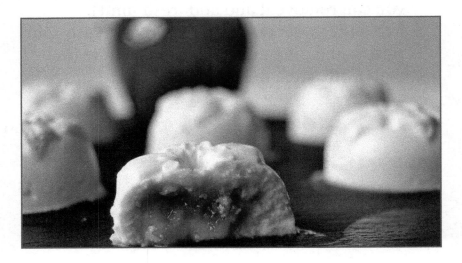

Servings 4

INGREDIENTS

- 150 g Ricotta
- 50 g Grated Parmesan
- 100 ml Whipping cream
- Gelatin 3 sheets
- Spicy jam for me, with peppers or tomatoes
-

PREPARATION

1. Soak the gelatin sheets in cold water.
2. Put the ricotta with the Parmesan and 25 ml of cream in a saucepan. Mix well and bring to a

boil over medium heat without stopping stirring.

3. As soon as it begins to boil, remove from the heat, drain the gelatin well, add it to the cream cheese and mix until the gelatin is completely dissolved. Let cool completely.

4. Whip the remaining cream and add it to the cream cheese and cream with enveloping movements from the bottom up.

5. Spread the cream obtained in a silicone mold filling the gaps halfway. Put some jam in the center and cover with more cream cheese.

6. Cover with cling film and put it in the fridge for at least two hours.

Pizza with burrata stracciatella

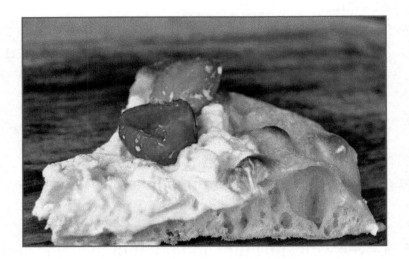

Servings 2

INGREDIENTS

For the burrata stracciatella
- 250 g Fresh mozzarella (2 units of 125)
- 200-250 ml Fresh cream for desserts
- Salt
- For the pizza dough (2 pizzas)
- 180 ml Water
- 2 g Fresh yeast
- 180 g Strength flour
- 80 g White flour
- Oil see
- 6 g Salt
- Candied tomatoes
- Stracciatella

- Basil

For the Stracciatella

- Take the mozzarella and go peeling it as if it were an onion, with a lot of patience you have to remove very thin layers, when there are no more layers you try to remove the threads and put them in a taper.
- Add the cream until covered, do not overdo it, limit yourself to what is essential.
- Salt fix.
- Let it rest in the refrigerator for 12-24 hours.
-

PREPARATION

1. Take the dough out of the refrigerator 5-10 hours before preparing the pizza and divide the dough into two balls (do not knead again, handle the dough as little as possible), sprinkle them well with flour, both below and above, cover them with a cloth and Let them rise at room temperature.
2. Roll out the dough using only your fingertips in a round shape and the size of your skillet.
3. Heat a pan over the fire and when it is very hot put the pizza base, add a few drops of oil on the surface and cook over medium heat until the base is golden and crisp.
4. Now put the pan in the highest part of the oven with the grill on and very hot, a couple of

minutes will be enough for the pizza to be golden brown.

5. Take out of the oven and add the stracciatella, some candied tomatoes, some basil leaves and serve.

Sweet and sour pumpkin

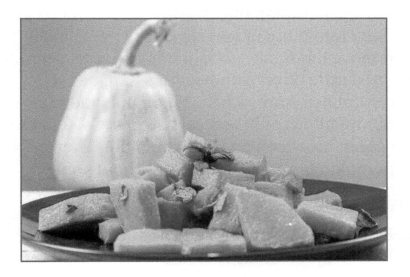

Serving: 4

INGREDIENTS

- 800 g Pumpkin
- 100 ml Vinegar (apple or wine, depending on your tastes)
- Sugar 2 teaspoons of coffee
- Oil ve cb
- Salt
- Garlic 1 clove
- Fresh mint 1 a bunch

PREPARATION

1. Cut the pumpkin into 0.5-1 cm slices, then cut them into more or less regular pieces. Finally, remove the skin (once cut it is easier to clean).
2. Put a little olive oil to heat in a pan, half a centimeter more or less. When hot, add the pumpkin pieces in several batches. Cook until golden brown on one side, then flip. The pumpkin has to be done but without going overboard, because if you do it, it falls apart (I like it to be firm).
3. Reserve on a plate and add a little salt.
4. Put vinegar and sugar in a glass. Stir until the sugar is completely dissolved.
5. Remove most of the oil from the pan, leave only 2-3 tablespoons (better if you use clean oil), add a peeled garlic clove and cook over medium heat until golden.
6. Then remove it from the oil.
7. Add the fried pumpkin, sauté a little and add the vinegar. Let it evaporate by sautéing from time to time.
8. Let the pumpkin rest for a few hours before serving (better a whole day), keep it with the oil from the last cooking. Serve it cold with some fresh mint leaves.

Fried calzone

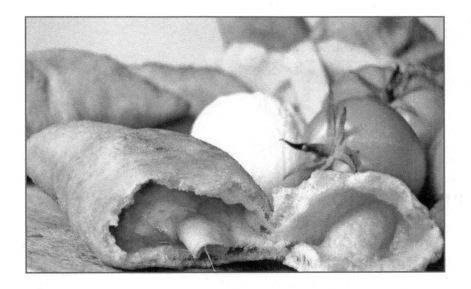

Serving: 4

INGREDIENT

For the mass
- 250 g Wheat flour
- 250 g W360 strength flour from El amasadero
- 125 g Milk
- 5 g Fresh yeast (long leavened 16-24 hours) or 15 g (short leavened 4-5 hours)
- 100-120 g Water
- Egg 1
- Butter at room temperature 25 g
- 10 g Sugar
- 25 g Salt

For the filling
- 200 g Tomato sauce
- 250 g Mozzarella
- 100g Cooked ham
- Oregano
- Basil
- Salt
- 700 ml oil for frying
-

PREPARATION

1. Sift the flours.
2. Put the yeast in a bowl and dissolve it with the milk, 100 g of water and the sugar, beating with a fork.
3. Add 150 g of flour, beat with a fork for a couple of minutes, like a tortilla.
4. Beat an egg, add half to the previous preparation (the other half save it for the preparation of the calzone) along with salt and butter, mix well with the fork until everything is well incorporated.
5. Add the remaining flour, mix first with the fork and then with your hands, turn the dough over on the counter and begin to knead like a pizza (if necessary add 10-20 ml of water) until you get a homogeneous dough, elastic and not too soft.
6. If you prepare the dough for the same day, divide it into small balls of about 50 g, put them

on a well-spaced tray, cover with a kitchen towel and leave it to ferment for 4-5 hours.

7. If you prepare the dough overnight (my favorite option) put it in a bowl, leave it at room temperature for an hour, and then put it in the refrigerator until the morning of the next day. Remove the dough from the bowl and without

8. Handling it too much, make small balls, put them on a well-spaced tray, cover with a kitchen cloth and let it rest in a warm place for 4 hours.

Eggplant caponata

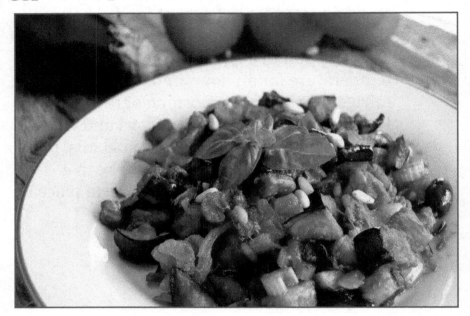

Servings 4

INGREDIENTS

- 800 g Eggplants
- Celery 4 stalks
- 1 large onion
- 1 tablespoon capers
- 3 tablespoons black olives
- 250 g Passata di pomodoro or crushed tomato
- 20 g Pine nuts
- 100 ml white wine vinegar
- Sugar 1 tablespoon
- Basil

- Salt
- Extra virgin olive oil
-

PREPARATION

1. Cut the aubergines into cubes, put them in a paste, salt evenly and let it rest for an hour so that the aubergines release the liquid and lose bitterness.
2. After this time, put the aubergines under the tap so that they release the excess salt. Drain them well and then dry them with a cloth.
3. Cut the stalks of the celery and onion, prepare a glass with vinegar and sugar.
4. In a frying pan, heat the oil and when it is ready, fry the aubergine cubes until golden brown. Take out of the oil and put them on top of a steel strainer so that they release the excess oil. Set aside on a plate.
5. When you finish with the aubergines, remove some of the oil, about half, and fry the onion and celery for about 3 minutes.
6. Add the olives, capers and lastly the pine nuts, fry a couple more minutes.
7. Add the tomato, mix, let it cook for a couple more minutes and then add the glass of vinegar with sugar that you had prepared at the beginning.
8. Let it evaporate and cook for about 5 minutes.

9. Now add the aubergine cubes, mix everything and let it cook together for another minute. Serve warm or cold. It is a dish that is best savored the day after it has been prepared.

Salmon carpaccio with citrus scent

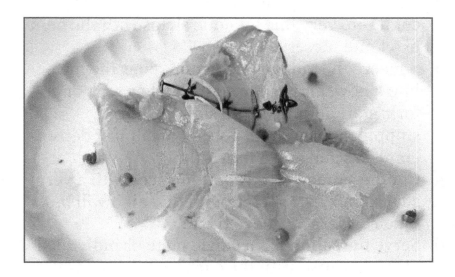

Servings 6

INGREDIENTS

- 500 g Fresh salmon
- Small orange 1
- Small lemon 1
- Extra virgin olive oil
- Pink pepper
- Salt

PREPARATION

1. With fresh and raw salmon

2. Freeze the salmon for at least 24 hours, then to defrost it, put it in the refrigerator.
3. Grate some of the citrus peel with a grater or cut it into very fine julienne strips with the help of a knife. Reserve them.
4. Squeeze the orange and lemon, pour the juice into a bowl and beat well with a few rods or a fork, start adding the oil slowly without stopping to beat until you get an almost dense emulsion and add a little salt.
5. Cut the salmon into very thin slices with a very sharp knife, if you start with the tail it will be much easier to remove them.
6. Serve the salmon in a single plate or individual plates, garnish with the citrus emulsion (as if you were to dress a salad) and a little pink pepper. Let stand 20 minutes before serving.
7. Garnish with the zest of the citrus peel.
8. With marinated salmon
9. The day before marinate the salmon following.

Glazed onions

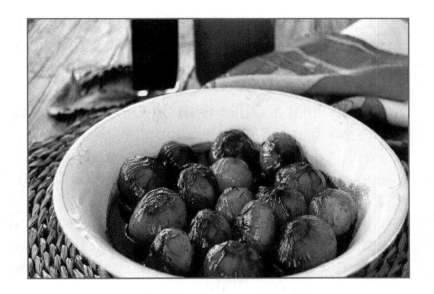

Serving: 4

INGREDIENTS

- 500 g French onions or shallots
- 150 ml Balsamic vinegar of Modena
- 100 ml Water
- Honey 3 tablespoons
- Butter 1 nut or 4 tablespoons oil
- Laurel 2 leaves
- Salt

PREPARATION

1. Clean the onions and put them in a bowl with water, Modena vinegar and honey. Stir well and if you are not in a hurry let it rest for half an hour.
2. Lightly heat a skillet with the oil or butter and the bay leaves. Add the onions with all the liquid where they have been marinated and cook over medium heat with the lid on for 10 minutes.
3. After time, remove the lid, add a little salt and continue cooking over medium heat for 25-30 minutes (depending on the size of the onions) until the cooking liquid is somewhat dense (keep in mind that when it cools it thickens more) .
4. Serve the glazed onions as an appetizer or side to a meat dish. To my taste cold they are much richer.

Cream of cheese and dried tomatoes

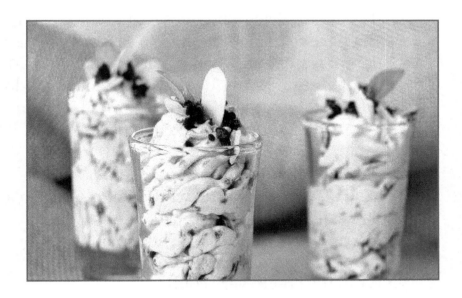

Servings 6

INGREDIENTS

- Dried tomatoes in oil 80 g or 60 g of dried tomatoes
- 200 g Ricotta cheese or other cream cheese
- 120 g Whipping cream
- Fresh basil 10 leaves
- Black pepper
- 30 g Rolled almonds
- Vinegar (optional)

PREPARATION

1. If you have dried tomatoes that are not in oil, you have to blanch them first. Put in a pot half a liter of water and when it starts to boil add 20 ml of vinegar. Wait for it to boil again and add the dried tomatoes. Cook for 5 minutes, then drain and pat dry with kitchen paper. Let it cool.
2. Put the tomatoes in a robot together with 6 basil leaves and mash giving a couple of strokes. You can also chop them with a knife. With Thermomix 7 sec. vel. 6. The tomato must be chopped and not made into a cream.
3. Whip the cream very cold.
4. Put the chopped tomatoes in a bowl (reserve a tablespoon to decorate the glasses) add the cheese and a pinch of pepper, mix well. With Thermomix put the cheese in the glass with the tomatoes and mix 4 sec. vel. 3.
5. Add the whipped cream and mix it gently. Let it rest in the refrigerator for half an hour.
6. While toasting the almonds in a pan.
7. Put the cream of cheese and tomatoes in a pastry bag with a star tip and distribute the cream into 6 glasses. Decorate each portion with the chopped dried tomatoes that you have set aside, the toasted almonds and chopped basil leaves (if they are small, put one in each glass).

Rice croquettes

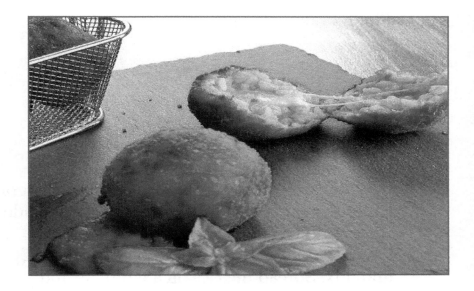

Servings 15

INGREDIENTS

- Rice 250g
- Eggs 2
- Saffron one strands
- Grated Parmesan cheese 50 g
- For the filling
- Mozzarella cheese 150 g
- Tomato crushed or fried 100g
- Minced meat 100g
- Onion 1/4
- White wine half a glass
- Salt

- To bread
- Bread crumbs
- Flour
- Eggs 2
- Salt
- 1/2 l olive oil for frying
-

PREPARATION

1. Cook the rice in the traditional way, put a pot of water to heat and as soon as it starts to boil add the rice and a few strands of saffron.
2. Drain the rice is ready, add the grated cheese and mix. Spread the rice on a flat plate and cool.
3. When it is cold add the eggs and mix well. If you want the simplest recipe like mine, without the meat, now also add the fried tomato and mix again, if you don't go to the next point to prepare the meat.
4. If you want to put the traditional filling, cook half a glass of peas.
5. In a pan with a little oil, fry the chopped onion, add the minced meat and fry until golden brown, add the white wine and evaporate. Finally add the crushed tomato, a pinch of salt and cook for about 10 minutes and that's it. Now add the peas, mix and that's it.
6. It is time to prepare the balls. If you put the meat and the peas you will have to make a

bigger ball. Take a tablespoon of dough and put it in the palm of your hand, flatten it with the help of the spoon and put the filling, first the meat (if you are going to put it in) and then the mozzarella. Close the ball well so that nothing comes out. You will get about 15 balls

7. It is time to pass them through flour, beaten egg and breadcrumbs.
8. Heat the oil to fry them. If possible try to cover at least half of the oil. Better to use a taller and smaller frying pan so as not to waste a lot of oil. Fry them for 2-3 minutes over medium high heat and stir them so that they brown evenly. When they are ready, put them on top of a steel rack to release the excess oil and then put them on kitchen paper.
9. They are ready to eat, better if hot. You can accompany them with a little fried tomato or just eat them like that.

Potato croquettes

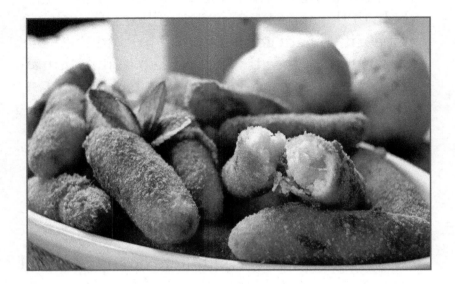

Servings 4

INGREDIENTS

- 500 g Potatoes
- 80 g Grated Parmesan cheese or cured sheep cheese
- 1 Egg
- Mint and parsley various leaves
- Salt
- To batter (optional)
- 2 whites Eggs
- Bread crumbs
- Salt
- Oil go to fry.

PREPARATION

1. Put the potatoes to cook in plenty of water until they are tender (check by pricking them with a fork). Peel them and pass them through a puree raisin or potato masher while they are still hot. Then let it cool.
2. Add finely chopped grated cheese, egg, salt, mint and parsley to the potatoes.
3. Mix well with your hands and let it rest for about 10 minutes.
4. Take small portions of dough and start to form the croquettes, the traditional ones have that classic elongated shape.
5. Now if you like them crunchier, you can coat it by first passing them in beaten egg white with a pinch of salt and then in breadcrumbs or you can also fry them as is.
6. Fry them in abundant oil, look very hot, they must be completely covered by the oil. Do not turn it over until it has first been well browned on one side.
7. Serve them still hot and you'll see how they will disappear. They are also delicious cold even if they are no longer crunchy.

Cauliflower and vegetable salad with a sweet and sour touch

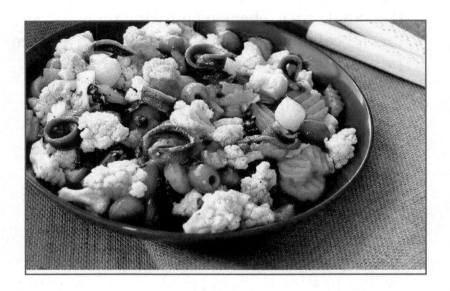

Servings 6

INGREDIENTS

- 750 g Cauliflower (so that we have about 500 g clean)
- 150 g Cucumber
- 1 small red pepper
- 100 g Carrots
- 1 tablespoon capers
- Anchovies 15 fillets
- 150 g Pickled onions
- 150 g Pitted olives
- 2 liters Water

- 250 g Sugar
- 250 g White wine vinegar
- 100 g Salt
- Pepper
- Oil see
-

PREPARATION

1. Wash the cauliflower and cut it so that we only have the little trees.
2. Wash and cut the other vegetables into 1/2 cm slices. The cucumber I leave it with the skin while the carrot I hair it.
3. Put the water in a pot along with vinegar, salt and sugar.
4. When the cauliflower comes to a boil and cooks for 5-6 minutes, it should be crisp. Drain it with a slotted spoon and put it in a bowl.
5. Cook the other vegetables at the same time in the same water for 3 minutes, drain them and let them cool with the cauliflower.
6. Put all the vegetables that you have cooked in a bowl.
7. Add pickled onions, capers, olives, and anchovy fillets. Season with olive oil, pepper and eventually salt.
8. The cauliflower and vegetable salad is ready, enjoy it cold.

Focaccia barese with tomatoes

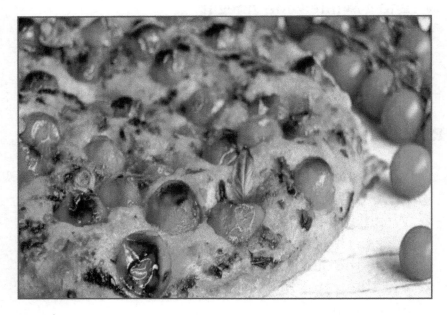

Serving: 4

INGREDIENTS

- 150 g W360 strength flour from El amasadero
- 100 g Rimacinata durum wheat semolina from El amasadero
- 60 g Cooked potato
- 3 g Fresh pressed baker's yeast
- 180 ml Water
- Oil ve 25 g + for the tomatoes and the source
- 7 g Salt
- 250-300 g Cherry tomatoes
- Tomato sauce or crushed tomato 2 tablespoons
- Oregano

PREPARATION

1. Mash the cooked potato with a masher or mashed raisin and put it in a bowl.
2. Add water, yeast and mix very well with a fork until the yeast and potato are dissolved (if there are lumps of potato you can use a robot so that it is well dissolved). Add the oil.
3. Add the strength flour and mix well with a fork for 1 minute. Beat the mixture as if it were an omelette so that the dough incorporates air.
4. Add salt and wheat semolina. Mix first with a fork, then grease your hands with oil and knead a little until you get a homogeneous appearance. The dough will be quite sticky.
5. Wash your hands. Spread the countertop with a little oil, pour the dough on top and make 4 folds (in the photos I have been missing the fold from bottom to top). Cover the dough with plastic wrap and let it rest for 15-20 minutes. Repeat this step at least 3 times with intervals of 15-20 minutes, do not forget to grease your hands with oil. You will see how each time your dough becomes more manageable and elastic (although it will always remain a bit sticky).
6. Spread a large tapper with oil, add the dough, cover it and let it rest for 1 hour at room temperature before putting it in the refrigerator. Let it rise in cold for 12 hours. After that time, take the dough out of the

refrigerator an hour before starting to spread the focaccia.

7. While dividing the tomatoes in half, put them on a plate and squash them a little so that they release liquid. Add salt, plenty of oregano, tomato sauce or crushed tomato and oil. Stir well.
8. Spread around dish between 26-32 cm in diameter. Pour the dough into the mold without barely touching it. Smear your hands with oil and spread the dough barely touching it with your fingertips.
9. Sprinkle the tomatoes and the accompanying juice on top. Slightly sink the tomatoes by gently squeezing with your fingers. Add a thread of oil on top and let the focaccia stand for another hour. Bake in a hot oven at 250° C for 20-25 minutes. The surface of the focaccia must be somewhat toasted (not burned), especially its edges must be crisp.
Serve it hot, warm or cold, it will always be a delight. It is the perfect recipe for snacking, to share with friends at your dinners or on the beach.

Focaccia with cherry tomatoes

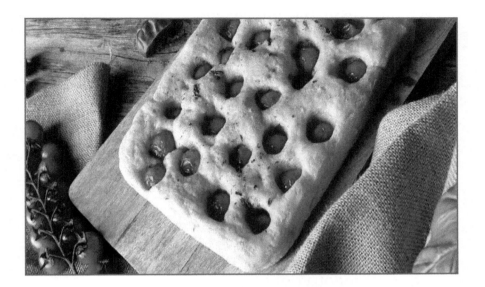

Servings 4

INGREDIENTS

- 300 g Flour
- 210 g Water
- 10 g baker's yeast
- Extra virgin olive oil
- 10 cherry tomatoes
- Salt
- Oregano
- 1 teaspoon coffee sugar

PREPARATION

1. We put the water, the yeast and the tip of a teaspoon of sugar in a glass and dissolve. In a bowl we will put the flour, form a volcano in the middle and add a teaspoon of salt.
2. Little by little we add the water with the yeast to the flour and we mix with the tips of the fingers first and then with the whole hand until we have finished the water.
3. We pass the dough on the counter and begin to knead for at least 5 minutes.
4. Add 3 charades of extra virgin oil and continue kneading for another 3 minutes until obtaining a homogeneous dough.
5. We grease a bowl with oil and deposit our dough. We cover with transparent film.
6. We let it rest for an hour.
7. While we cut the cherry tomatoes in half and season them with salt and oregano and a good drizzle of oil. With the help of a fork we are crushing them a little so that they release a little juice.
8. After the hour of rest of our dough we take a baking tray we spread it
9. with oil and sprinkle with a little salt. Take the bowl with the dough and make it
10. Gently slide into pan, use fingers to distribute evenly, being careful not to lose air from the dough.

11. We pour the tomatoes with all the liquid on top of our dough and spread over the surface. The tomatoes will have to be cut side down, in contact with the dough. Then press it gently. Let rise another hour and a half hours or until the tomatoes are slightly sunk in the dough.
12. Bake with a hot oven at 200 degrees for 30-40 minutes and until the surface turns a golden color
13. Remove from the oven and immediately splash, with the help of your fingers, the surface of the focaccia with a little water. Let stand 10 minutes.

Quick focaccia with cheese and pesto

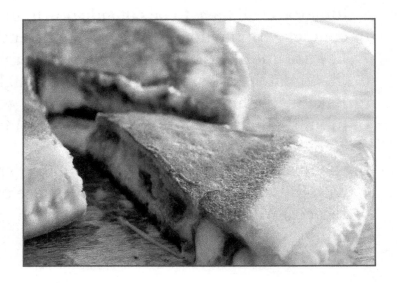

Serving: 4

INGREDIENTS

- 125 g Durum wheat semolina flour
- 125 g Wheat flour (or just 250 g of wheat flour)
- Medium sachet baker's yeast powder (or 15 g fresh yeast)
- 150 ml Milk or water approximately (varies according to the type of flour)
- 1 teaspoon salt
- Extra virgin olive oil 3 tablespoons
- For the filling
- Striped mozzarella cheese (the one that comes in sachets)

- Emmental cheese
- 3 tablespoons basil pesto
-

PREPARATION

1. Dissolve the yeast in a little water.
2. Put the flours in a bowl, make a hole in the middle and first add the water with the dissolved yeast, mix well with your fingers and then add the rest of the water. Add the salt and continue kneading until there is no more loose dough.
3. Pass the dough on the counter, stretch it a little and add the oil.
4. Knead for a few minutes until you get a smooth, uniform and elastic texture.
5. Put the dough back in the bowl, cover with cling film and let it rest for 30-40 minutes and until the dough has doubled in volume.
6. When the dough is ready, divide it into two parts and stretch them in a circular shape with the help of a rolling pin.
7. Grease the base of a frying pan with oil (mine is 26 cm) and place a disk of dough, you can help yourself with the rolling pin to move it.
8. Distribute the cheeses on top, a little pesto and place the other disk of dough. Trim the remaining dough around the edges.

9. Cook over medium heat for approximately 8 minutes, check that it is done and turn it over. Cook another 4 minutes on the other side. The quick focaccia with cheese and pesto is ready, hot is when it is best

Italian style filled puff pastry, rustic leccese

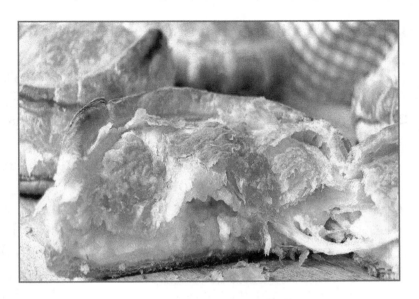

Servings 4

INGREDIENTS

- Puff pastry 3 rolls (for single portion or 2 for family)
- 75 ml Tomato-sauce
- 125 g Mozzarella
- 350 ml Milk at room temperature
- 50 g Flour
- 20 g Butter
- Pepper
- Nutmeg
- Salt
- Egg 1

PREPARATION

1. Put flour and butter in a saucepan, cook over medium low heat for 6-7 minutes without stopping stirring with a wooden spoon until you get a golden mixture.
2. Add a little milk, mix with the spoon until it is absorbed and then add more, always little by little. Do not add more if the previous dose has not been absorbed to avoid clumping.
3. Add salt, pepper, nutmeg and cook for about 7 minutes over medium heat, stirring constantly, until you get a fairly thick béchamel. Let it cool. With thermomix: put butter and flour in the glass 10 min 120° or varoma speed 2. Add milk, salt, pepper and nutmeg 7 min 90° speed 4. Let cool. Once cold, if you take it with a spoon, it should be compact.
4. preparation single-portion rustic assembly
5. Open the puff pastry rolls and remove from each sheet some discs of about 11-12 cm in diameter (12 discs in total come out).
6. Take 4 of them and cut a smaller disk inside to form a ring that is 1 cm wide (as in the photos).
7. Put vegetable paper on the baking tray, place 4 discs on top and brush them with beaten egg.
8. Place in the middle of each 2-3 tablespoons of cold bechamel, 1 tablespoon of tomato and the diced mozzarella. Try to make the filling in the shape of a squashed mountain.

9. Cover each unit with another disk and glue the edges of the two bases well with the help of a fork.

10. Brush the entire surface with egg and place the ring on top so that the mountain of filling is in the center. Gently squash the base and brush with egg again.

11. Bake in a hot oven at 200° C for 25-30 minutes, do not overcook them because otherwise they will open and the filling will come out.

12. Let them sit for about 15 minutes at room temperature before eating them.

13. Rustic family setting

14. Spread a sheet on the baking tray covered with greaseproof paper, brush the edges with beaten egg.

15. Put tomato, béchamel and mozzarella in the middle. Place the other sheet on top and close the edges well.

16. Another option is to make 1 Italian filled puff pastry with each sheet, in this case you will have to fill it following the previous steps and then you will close it in a book.

17. Bake in a hot oven at 200°C for 25-30 minutes, do not overcook them because otherwise they will open.

    Let them sit for about 15 minutes at room temperature before eating them.

Pittule" or fried dough

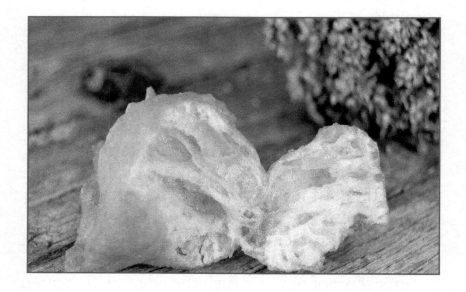

Servings 3

INGREDIENT

- 10 g Pressed yeast
- 270 g Water
- 400 g Wheat flour
- Salt
- Optional padding
- 1 tablespoon capers
- Anchovies 8 anchovies
- To fry
- Extra virgin olive oil

PREPARATION

1. In a large bowl, dissolve the yeast in the water.
2. Sift the flour and add it to the water little by little, mixing with a spoon.
3. Once you have added all the flour, continue mixing vigorously for a couple more minutes. It will be a sticky dough.
4. If you want them to have more flavor add anchovies cut in half and capers, mix well until well incorporated.
5. Put it to proof in a place away from the draft for at least 2-3 hours until it has almost tripled its volume (before and after photos).
6. In a frying pan, heat plenty of oil with a piece of lemon peel.
7. When the skin will be golden, it will be time to pour the dough.
8. Take two spoons and spread them in oil, take with them small portions of dough and then drop them in the hot oil. Cook for 1 minute on each side until golden brown. Drain on kitchen paper, then serve while still hot.

Mussels au gratin

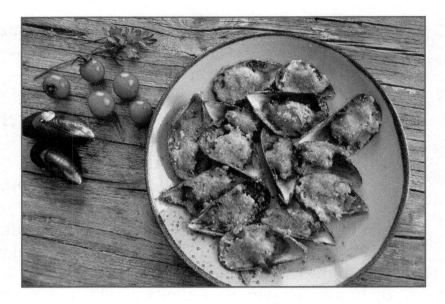

Servings 3

INGREDIENTS

- 1 kg Mussels
- Bread crumbs
- 50 g Grated sheep's cheese or parmesan
- Cherry tomatoes (optional) 2 units
- Garlic a clove
- Parsley
- Pepper
- Oregano

PREPARATION

1. We wash the mussels well.
2. We eliminate the filaments that protrude between the two shells by pulling down.
3. We position on top of the baking tray that we are going to use (so as not to lose the water that comes out of the mussels), we take a pointed knife and hold the mussel with our left hand, keeping its oval part closer to. us. We will push the shell from above to the right and with the index finger we will push the shell from below to the left. If the mussels are very fresh, we will hear a click that indicates that the mussel is no longer sealed.
4. Now we can insert the tip of the knife between the two shells. We incline the knife until its tip touches the shell above. We move the knife towards us always keeping the tip up so as not to destroy the mollusk. We put the blade of the knife vertically and it is already open.
5. With the help of your hands you can finish opening it to be able to remove the shell from above and throw it away. We have our mussel ready
6. Preparation of the mussels
7. While we are opening the mussels we are placing them one very close to the other without overlapping.
8. When we have them all, sprinkle with a thin layer of grated cheese and bread. Then we will

put the chopped cherry tomatoes and garlic, pepper, parsley and oregano, and sprinkle with cheese and bread again.

9. Serve hot, warm or cold.

Eggplant jam

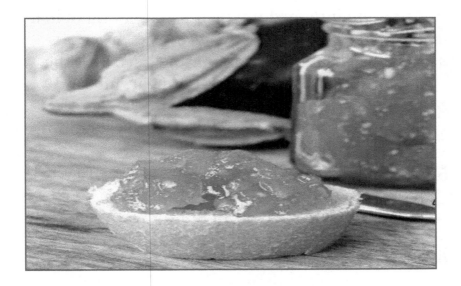

Servings 3

INGREDIENTS

- 500 g Eggplants
- 400 g Sugar
- Medium lemon
- Medium orange
- 15 g Fresh ginger

PREPARATION

1. Scratch the skins from the citrus fruits and set them aside.

2. Wash the aubergines, cut the top and peel them leaving part of the skin.
3. Cut them into medium pieces and put them in a bowl.
4. Squeeze the lemon and pour the juice over the aubergines, mix well. Add the sugar, mix and pour everything into a pot. Add the reserved citrus peels and cook 10 minutes over medium heat, stirring occasionally.
5. While squeezing the orange and grating the ginger. Add them to the aubergines and cook over low heat for about 15 minutes, stirring often.
6. Pour the still hot aubergine jam into previously boiled jars, close them and turn them upside down until cold. To pasteurize the jars, wrap them in kitchen cloths and boil them for 20 minutes. Do not remove it from the water until it is cold, then pat it dry and store it in a dark place.

Chilli jam

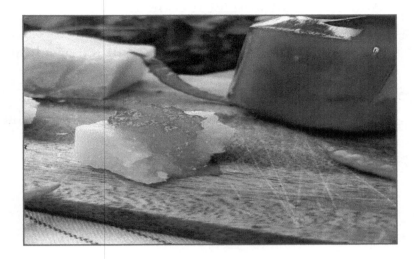

Servings 3

INGREDIENTS
- 5-10 g Fresh chillies
- 500 g Red pepper
- 200 g Sugar

PREPARATION

1. Wash the peppers and chillies. Remove the seeds from the peppers but not from the chillies.
2. Cut the peppers and chillies into small pieces.
3. Put everything in a well covered saucepan and cook over medium heat for 7 minutes.

4. Blend with a blender, I prefer not to leave it pureed, I like it to be chunky.
5. Add the sugar and let it cook another 10 minutes over medium heat uncovered (if it splashes a lot at first, put a lid but leave a hole for it to evaporate)
6. When the jam starts to get a little honeyed it will be ready. Package in previously boiled glass jars, cover and turn over until cold.

Pizza snack

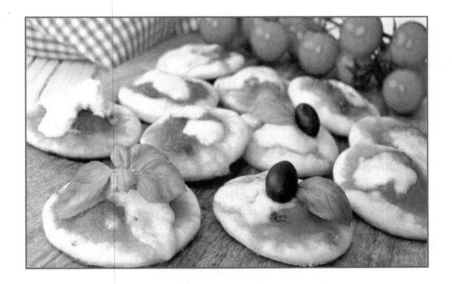

Serving: 4

INGREDIENTS

- 220 g Pizza flour (with built-in yeast)
- 250 g Greek yogurt without sugar 2 cups
- 5 g Salt
- On top of the pizzas
- 50 g Tomato sauce
- Mozzarella 1
- Oregano
- Salt

PREPARATION

1. Put all the pizza ingredients in a bowl, mix first with a fork and then knead with your hands until you get a homogeneous dough. If it is sticky add a little more flour. With Thermomix put all the ingredients in the glass and program 1 minute spike mode.
2. Transfer the dough to the counter, sprinkle both the dough and the work surface with flour. Roll out the dough to a thickness of 3mm or so.
3. With a glass you take out the mini pizzas. Knead the leftover dough again and take out more pizzas.
4. Put the mini pizzas on a baking tray lined with greaseproof paper and add in the center of each a little tomato sauce seasoned with oregano and salt.
5. Bake at 180° for 5 minutes, remove from the oven and add the mozzarella. Bake again for 10 more minutes.

Cheese mousse with caramelized pears and ham

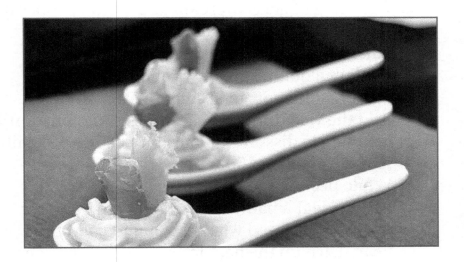

Servings 3

INGREDIENTS

- 120 g Parmigiano cheese
- 200 ml cooking cream
- White pepper
- 1 Gelatin sheets
- 1 Pear conference
- 1 nut butter
- Serrano ham 2 slices

PREPARATION

1. Soak the gelatin in cold water.
2. Put 100 g of cheese, cream and a little pepper in a saucepan, stir until all the ingredients are amalgamated.
3. Cook in a double boiler without stopping stirring until you get a smooth cream.
4. Add the well drained gelatin sheet and mix until completely dissolved. Pour into a bowl and chill in the fridge for 1 hour.
5. While peeling the pear and cut it into small cubes. Heat a pan with a small knob of butter over low heat and when it is melted add the pear. Turn up the heat to the highest and sauté from time to time until it takes on a golden and transparent appearance. Do not stir with a spoon because it will be pureed.
6. Heat a frying pan (without oil) and put teaspoons of cheese on top. It has to be in very thin layers. When the cheese starts to brown and melt, roll it up with a spatula. When they are ready, reserve them.
7. Prepare the final dish. Place a little caramelized pear in a ceramic spoon (you can also use disposable spoons), put the cheese mousse in a pastry bag and distribute it in each portion.
8. Cut the ham loaches into small strips and roll them to form a rose. Place it on the mousse.
9. Finish the cheese mousse with caramelized pears and ham with the crunchy cheese.

Baci di dama

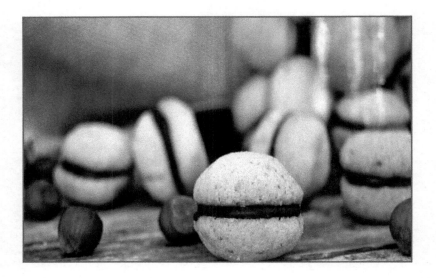

Servings 50

INGREDIENTS

- 200 g roasted hazelnuts (or almonds)
- 200 g Icing sugar
- 180 g Cold butter
- 220 g Flour
- 150 g Dark chocolate
-

PREPARATION

1. Crush the hazelnuts with 50 g of sugar using a food processor. If it is small, divide them into several batches, distributing the sugar between

them. It is important not to heat the flour that is obtained, so grind with brief turbo strokes.

2. Put the remaining 150 g of sugar and the cold butter in a bowl. Work the dough with the tips of your fingers until the two ingredients are mixed. Be careful not to heat the dough.

3. Add flour and ground hazelnuts. First you will get a grainy mixture, then knead until you get a compact and homogeneous dough. Shape it into a rectangle 1.5 - 2 cm thick, wrap it in plastic wrap and let it rest in the refrigerator for at least 4-5 hours (I prepare it the night before).

4. Take the dough, cut it first into strips and then into cubes. Weigh each one of them, they will all have to be the same, about 7 g (the original is 3 g). Mold them gently with the palm of your hands to get small balls. Place them well spaced apart on a parchment-lined cookie sheet. When you finish, put the entire tray in the refrigerator and let it rest for at least one hour.

5. Heat the oven to 150° C. When it is hot, put the tray just taken out of the refrigerator and cook for about 20 minutes until the cookies are golden brown. Once ready, take them out of the oven and wait until they are very cold.

6. Find the perfect pair of each cookie to mount the lady kisses.

7. Melt the chocolate in a double boiler or microwave. Heat it to the bare minimum. Then stir with a spatula until it becomes a little thick.

8. Helping you with a spoon, place a little chocolate in the center of one of the two halves of the bacio di dama. Make sure the chocolate is in the center without reaching the edges. Allow the chocolate time to settle well and while you distribute it in a cookie of each pair.

9. When you finish distributing the chocolate, take the other pair from each kiss and place it on top of the chocolate cookie, do not squeeze. Wait a few seconds and try to balance it so that the top cookie stays centered. Don't move the lady kisses until the chocolate has hardened.

10.   Store the baci di dama in a tightly closed jar, they hold up very well for a couple of weeks.

Biancomangiare, dessert with almond milk

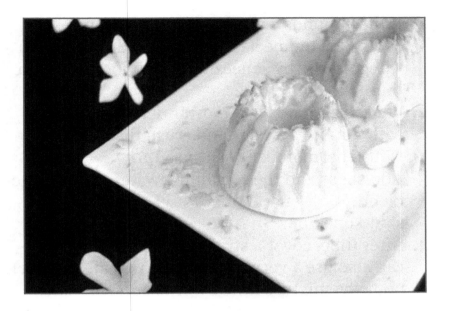

Servings 5

INGREDIENTS

- For the almond milk
- 200 Raw almonds 200
- 900 ml Water 900 ml
- Sugar 40 g
- For the biancomangiare
- 500 ml Almond milk
- Lemon 1 (skin only)
- 30 g Sugar
- 45 g Cornstarch
- 30 g Rolled almonds

PREPARATION

1. If the almonds are with skin, soak them overnight and peel them the next day. The skin will go easily by squeezing the almond between thumb and forefinger.
2. Put the almonds in a mortar or food processor with 400 ml of water and crush them finely. With Thermomix 25 sec speed 10.
3. Add sugar and the remaining water, continue to blend. With Thermomix 10 sec speed 10. Let stand one hour.
4. After time, cover a strainer with a gauze (you can also use a very narrow mesh metal strainer) pour the mixture little by little and stir with a spoon so that the milk is filtered. When all the milk has been filtered, press the gauze over the ground almonds to remove all the milk that remains.
5. The almond milk is ready, if you do not use it at the moment, keep it in the refrigerator for a maximum of 4-5 days. You can use the ground almonds to make an almond slush or for sponge cakes Biancomangiare
6. Dissolve the cornstarch in a glass with 100 ml of almond milk
7. Grate the lemon peel and put it in a saucepan along with 400 ml of milk and the sugar. Heat over medium heat for a couple of minutes. With Thermomix 2 min 100° speed 2.

8. Filter the milk with a strainer where you have dissolved the cornstarch and add it to the milk that you are heating.
9. Stir vigorously over medium heat until the milk thickens and starts to boil a little. With Thermomix 4 min 100° speed 2.

   Pour the biancomangiare into silicone molds previously wet with water and let it rest in the refrigerator for a few hours.

   Before serving, heat a pan and lightly toast the sliced almonds. Sprinkle each serving with the sliced and toasted almonds. You already have the dessert ready to serve it.

Lemon and almond cake, also with Thermomix

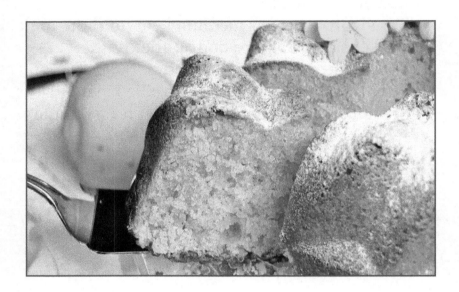

Servings 6

INGREDIENTS

- 120 g Pastry flour El amasadero (unleavened)
- 75 Potato starch or cornstarch
- 150 g Finely ground almonds
- 200 g Butter
- 240 g Icing sugar
- 6 fresh organic lemons (6 skin and 1 juice)
- 3 size L Eggs
- 150 ml Milk
- 1 pod Vanilla (or vanilla extract)
- Yeast for dessert (Royal type) 1 sachet

- 3 g Salt
-

PREPARATION

1. Grate the skin of the lemons.
2. Put it in a bowl with room temperature butter and the seeds of the vanilla bean (or extract). Mix with a spatula and let it rest for about 20 minutes, stirring from time to time.
3. After time, add icing sugar and salt, work the dough with electric rods until you get a voluminous dough.
4. Add the eggs one by one and assemble the dough always using electric rods. Do not add the next egg until the previous one has been completely absorbed. When you finish with the eggs, keep riding with the rods for a couple more minutes.
5. Sift the flour and put it in a clean bowl with the yeast, the potato starch or cornstarch and the ground almonds. Stir with a spoon so that they are well mixed.
6. Add 4 tablespoons of flour to the butter mixture and stir.
7. Add the milk in a thread without stopping to beat with the rods.
8. Finally add the remaining flour mixture and continue beating until you get a homogeneous dough.

9. Finally add the lemon juice and incorporate it gently with a spatula making enveloping movements from the bottom up.
Butter a mold and sprinkle it with flour. Pour the cake batter inside and spread it evenly with a spatula. Bake in a hot oven at 160° C for about 1 hour. To see if it's ready, do the toothpick test. Leave the cake in the oven turned off and ajar for another 10 minutes. Unmold once cold. If you want you can sprinkle it with icing sugar (only when it is totally cold).

Apple cake

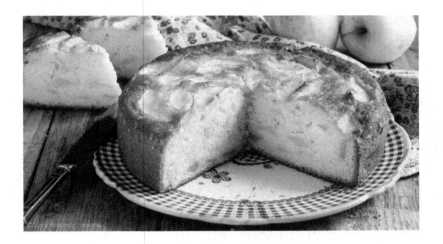

Servings 8

INGREDIENTS

- 500 g Organic apples
- Medium organic lemon
- 3 size L Eggs
- 180 g Sugar
- 90 g Ve mild or sunflower oil
- 330 g Flour
- 15 g Yeast for desserts (or an envelope)
- Powdered sugar to sprinkle.

PREPARATION

1. Peel half a lemon with a potato peeler, cut the apples into pieces eliminating the seeds and the peduncle (if the apples are not organic, it is better to peel them). Put the apple, lemon peel and lemon juice in a robot, blend everything until you get a puree.
2. Separate the yolks from the whites.
3. Mount the whites to snow until it makes the horns.
4. In another bowl, whip the yolks with the sugar for about 5 minutes until they become lighter and more voluminous. Add the oil and mix again.
5. Slowly pour the yolks into the egg whites bowl while stirring with the rods.
6. Add the applesauce and stir gently.
7. Sift the flour together with the yeast and add it to the other ingredients with gentle movements.
8. Butter a mold and sprinkle it with flour.
9. Pour the apple cake dough inside and bake in a hot oven at 180°C for 45 minutes. Perform the toothpick test to make sure it's done.
10. Unmold the cake only when it is cold and sprinkle with icing sugar.

Pumpkin and almond sponge cake

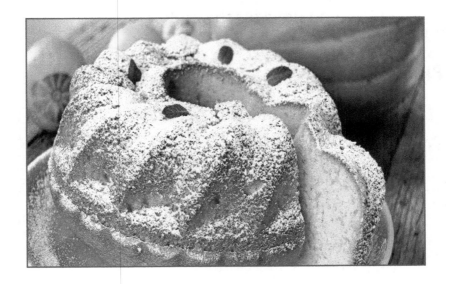

Servings 6

INGREDIENTS

- 250 g Pumpkin already clean 250 g
- 100 ml Sunflower oil or go smooth 100 ml
- 80 ml Milk 80 ml
- Eggs L 4
- 1 pinch salt
- 200 g Sugar 200 g
- 280 g Wheat flour 280 g
- 125 g Ground peeled almonds 125 g
- Orange peel
- Peel of half a lemon
- Rum or lemon or orange juice 4 tablespoons

- Yeast for desserts 1 sachet
- 2 tablespoons icing sugar (optional)
- Butter and flour for the mold
-

PREPARATION

1. Put chopped pumpkin, oil, milk, citrus peel, orange juice or rum in a food processor and finely grind everything. Reserve in a bowl.
2. Separate the yolks from the whites. Whip the yolks with 150 g of sugar until they triple in volume and are lighter in color.
3. Add the pumpkin cream to the yolks and mix very well.
4. Add flour, ground almonds, yeast and continue mixing.
5. Whip the egg whites with 50 g of sugar and a pinch of salt. Then add them to the previous mixture little by little using a spatula and making gentle movements from the bottom up.
6. Spread a bowl with butter, sprinkle it with flour, pour in the sponge dough and bake in a hot oven at 180° for 40-45 minutes. Do the toothpick test to see if it's ready. Once cold, remove the mold. If you want you can sprinkle with icing sugar.

Chocolate bonbons with Italian meringue

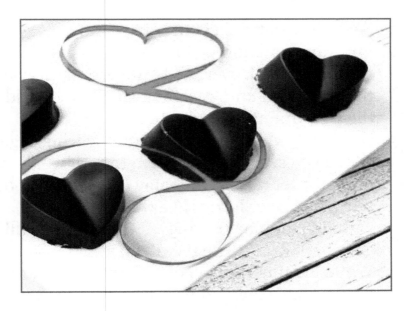

Servings 12

INGREDIENTS

- 130 g Egg whites (approximately those of 4 eggs L)
- 200 g Sugar
- 50 g icing sugar
- 1 sheet Gelatin
- 50 g Water
- Wafers 4 units (of the large round ones)
- 250 g 70% dark chocolate

PREPARATION

1. Soak the gelatin sheet in cold water.
2. Put water and 200 g of normal sugar in a saucepan. Cook over moderate heat to dissolve the sugar and until reaching 120° C then add the well-drained gelatin sheet.
3. In a bowl, whip the whites with the icing sugar. When you see that they begin to turn white but have not yet reached a foamy consistency, pour the syrup very slowly (in a thread) at 120° without stopping beating. At the end you will get a very firm meringue. Keep it in the fridge.
4. While melting the chocolate in the microwave or in a bain-marie. Pour some of the melted chocolate into a silicone mold and distribute it well with a spatula. Put the mold in the freezer for a couple of minutes and then distribute a little more chocolate (helping you with a spatula) to get a homogeneous layer of chocolate, which does not break when unmolding. Cover the chocolate mold well up to the edges and store in the refrigerator.
5. Cut the wafers to the shape of the bases of your molds.
6. When the chocolate molds have been very cold, fill them with the meringue until a little less than the edge. Top with the cut wafer and top with melted dark chocolate. Reserve in the refrigerator for 1 hour.

7. It is time to unmold, it is the most delicate phase. Peel the silicone mold from the chocolate meringue pralines a little by pulling the edges.
8. Take them out very carefully.
9. Once you have them out, remove any imperfections from the base with the tip of the knife. They are ready, I hope you like them!

Baci Perugina, chocolate and hazelnut bonbons

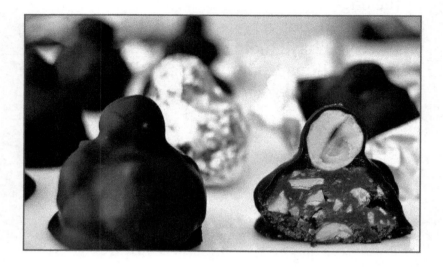

Servings 25

INGREDIENTS

- 100 g Milk chocolate
- 20 g Butter
- 100 g Hazelnut cream
- 100 g Roasted hazelnuts + 25 whole roasted hazelnuts
- 200 g 70% dark chocolate 200 g

PREPARATION

1. Chop the milk chocolate and butter, put them in a bowl and melt in a double boiler or in the microwave. In thermomix 5 min. 50° speed 1.
2. While chopping 100 g of hazelnuts with a knife, do not use a robot so that they are not too crumbled or powdered.
3. When the chocolate is ready add the hazelnut cream and the chopped hazelnuts. Mix with a spatula and put the bowl in the freezer for 15-20 minutes.
4. When the dough is cold, take a small portion and make a ball out of it, flatten it a little and place a whole hazelnut on top, pressing lightly.
5. Chop the dark chocolate and melt it in a double boiler, in the microwave or with a Thermomix for 5 min. 70° vel. 1.5. Then pour it into a glass.
6. Prick the base of the chocolate and hazelnut bonbons with a toothpick (this is the link of the video on Instagram) and dip the chocolate bar, when you take it out, let it drain for a few seconds and put the bon bon on top of a rack (better the rack of the greaseproof paper, so that it drains well). As you make all the chocolates, you will have little dark chocolate left, then continue dipping the base of the chocolates as you have done so far, then rest the chocolate on the rack and pour the dark chocolate on top.

7. When they have drained, take the chocolates by lifting them with two forks, without touching the sides, transfer them on baking paper and put them in the refrigerator until they harden.
8. While cutting aluminum foil into a 10x10 cm square, you paint some stars with an indelible pen, if you want to write a message on a strip of baking paper and wrap each chocolate bar.

Bon bon of dried fig ice cream

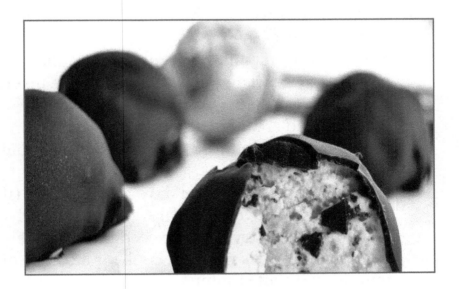

Servings 6

INGREDIENTS

- 580 g Whole milk
- 180 g Cream 35% fat
- 40 g Skimmed milk powder
- 5 g Locust bean gum
- 100 g White sugar
- 55 g Dextrose or 35 g invert sugar
- 80 g Dried figs
- 200 g Dark chocolate

PREPARATION

1. Grind the figs with a robot, it does not matter if there are pieces left.
2. Put locust bean gum, sugar, dextrose, milk powder in a bowl and mix well (if you use invert sugar add it in step 4).
3. Put milk and cream in a saucepan, heat over medium-low heat until it reaches 50° C without stopping to stir.
4. Add the powders that you have mixed before (if you use invert sugar add it now) and stir until reaching 80° C (try not to exceed them), once the temperature is reached, cook for a couple of minutes without stopping stirring.
5. Remove from the heat and add 50 g of chopped dried figs and using an immersion robot, grind everything very well.
6. Add the remaining 30 g of chopped figs and mix everything very well with just one epsatula.
7. When you finish, pour everything into a tapper and let it rest in the refrigerator for at least 6 hours.
8. Preparation of the mixture with Thermomix
9. Put the dried figs in the glass and crush 8 sec vel 8. Reserve in a bowl.
   Put in a bowl sugar, dextrose (if you use invert sugar add it in step 4), powdered milk and locust bean gum, mix everything very well. Without washing the glass add milk and cream, program 5 minutes 50° C vel. two.

10.　　Add the content of the bowl that you have prepared before (if you use invert sugar add it now) and program 5 minutes at 80° C vel. 2.5.
11. Add 50 g of dried figs 4 sec speed 5.
12. Add the remaining part of dried figs, stir with a spatula and pour everything into a tapper. Let it rest in the refrigerator for at least 6 hours.
13. Ice cream preparation
14. Take the ice cream mixture out of the refrigerator and mix very well with a few rods. Pour the preparation little by little into the refrigerator and butter for approximately 40 minutes.
15. Pour into a previously refrigerated tapper and put in the freezer for at least 1 hour.
16. You can already eat the dried fig ice cream but I advise you to continue with the recipe to try the chocolates.
17. Preparation of the fig ice cream bonbons
Put a plate in the freezer to chill. When the ice cream has acquired more consistency, take a half sphere of ice cream with an ice cream spoon and place it on the plate that you have cooled (better if you cover it with greaseproof paper). As soon as you have all the ice cream balls, put them back in the freezer for a couple of hours so that they are firm.
Put the chocolate in a glass and melt it in the microwave. Heat it to the minimum necessary, stirring often, try not to exceed 50 °C.

Take the ice cream scoops from the freezer, prick it with a wooden skewer or with a clothespin, and completely submerge it in the chocolate. Let it drain a little and turn the ice cream bon bon color on the vegetable film. Reheat the chocolate when you see it getting too cold. Put the chocolates in the freezer and let them rest for at least 10 minutes before serving. If you prepare the chocolates or ice cream overnight, remove them from the freezer 5 minutes before serving.

Sicilian brioche

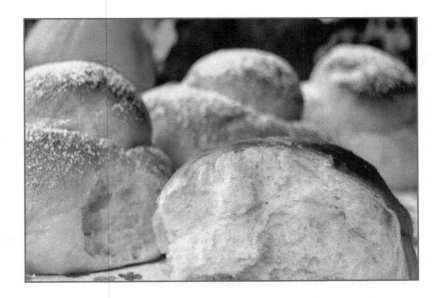

Servings 4

INGREDIENTS

- 170 ml Whole milk
- 5 g Fresh pressed yeast
- 500 g Strength flour
- Eggs 2
- 80-100 g White sugar
- Orange peel
- Peel of half a lemon
- 20 g Honey
- 5 g Salt
- 80 g Butter at room temperature
- To brush

- Yolk 1
- Milk
-

PREPARATION

1. In a large bowl put the milk at room temperature and the yeast, with the help of a fork beat well until the yeast is completely dissolved.
2. Sift the flour and add it to the milk, mix well with a spoon, it will be a loose and a little lumpy dough.
3. First add an egg, knead with your hands and when it is completely mixed add the other egg. Keep kneading until you get a homogeneous dough.
4. Grate the citrus peels and add them to the dough together with sugar, salt and honey. Knead for a few minutes until everything is well mixed and the dough begins to gather body and be elastic.
5. 5. Finally add the soft butter in small quantities, do not add the next dose if the first has not been fully adsorbed. Transfer the dough on the counter, knead for a few minutes until you get an elastic, shiny and homogeneous dough. If it is a bit sticky, smear the work surface and your hands with oil.

6. Put the dough in a plastic bowl, cover it with plastic wrap and let it rest in the refrigerator for 24-36 hours.
7. After the cold rest time has elapsed, the dough will have grown a little, take it out of the refrigerator and let it rest for a couple of hours in a warm place or in the oven with the light on.
8. How to prepare the dough with Thermo mix
9. Put the orange and lemon peel in the glass (peel them with a potato peeler) with 50 g of sugar and program 10 sec. vel. 10. If there are pieces of skin left, grind again for a few more seconds. Reserve in a bowl.
10. Without washing the glass, add the milk, yeast and mix for 10 sec. vel. 3.5.
11. Now add the previously sifted flour and mix 30 sec. vel 5. You will get a loose and somewhat lumpy dough.
12. Put the machine at spike speed while it is in motion, first add one egg and about 30 seconds later the second. Knead another 1 minute in herringbone mode.
13. Now add the crushed citrus peels with the sugar, the remaining sugar, the salt, the honey and program 2 minutes in spike mode.
14. Smear a little oil on the work surface and your hands.
15. Put the dough on the counter and divide it into 10 pieces of 80 g and another 10 of 10 g.
16. Take the large pieces and give it a round shape, you have to "roll" the dough as is done with the

pandoro put each hand to one side and at the base of the dough, then move one hand towards you and the other in the opposite direction several times, until the dough has a spherical and well homogeneous shape.

17. Give small pieces a round shape first and then tape one side.

18.   Now you have to assemble the two pieces, click the large ball with a finger where you will place the small ball on the side of the cone and press down hard. It is important that the ball is well nailed and stuck so that it does not fall during rest.

19. Place the brioches on a baking tray lined with greaseproof paper, cover them with cling film and let them rest until they double in size.

20.   Brush each brioche with a whipped yolk mixture, a little milk and bake in a hot oven at 180° C for 15-20 minutes and that's it. Once ready, let it cool on a rack.

21. Serve them as is, you can also dip them in milk, coffee, fill them with ice cream or Sicilian slushies.

Ricotta and orange fritters

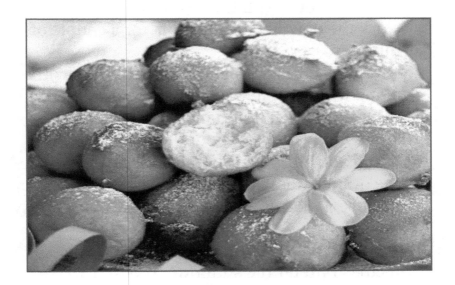

Servings 40

INGREDIENTS

- 250 g Ricotta cheese
- 120 g Sugar
- Medium orange 1 (skin and juice)
- 260-280 g Pastry flour from El amasadero
- 1 Egg
- 5 g Royal type yeast for desserts
- Oil for frying

PREPARATION

1. Put the ricotta with the sugar in a bowl and work the dough with a spatula for a couple of minutes.
2. Grate the orange peel and add it to the ricotta along with its squeezed juice. Mix very well.
3. Add beaten egg, flour, and yeast. Start by adding only 260 g of flour, if the dough is too liquid add a little more (it will depend on how the orange was). Mix very well with the spatula until you get a homogeneous and slightly sticky dough.
4. Heat in a pan with plenty of oil (for these recipes I prefer the sunflower). With two dessert spoons, take a little dough, the size of a small walnut, shape it (as is done with croquettes) and drop the dough in the hot oil. Fry for a couple of minutes over a low heat (I 7 out of 10 in my induction), so they will be golden brown and well done. Scoop out and drain on kitchen paper.
5. If you don't eat them freshly made once cold, you can sprinkle them with icing sugar.

Canestrelli, also with Thermomix

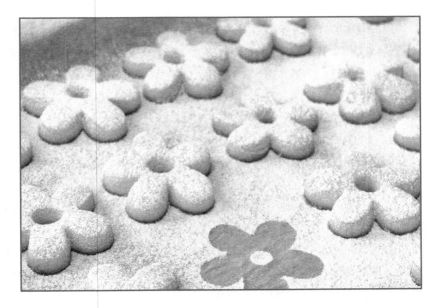

Servings 40

INGREDIENTS

- 120 g Glass sugar + 30 g to sprinkle
- 200 g Butter
- 200 g Wheat flour
- 100 Potato starch or cornstarch
- 1 or 2 small Large lemon
- 8 medium Eggs
- Salt

PREPARATION

1. Put the eggs to cook in a saucepan with water and let them boil for 8 minutes. When they are ready, put them in cold water and once cool, remove the peel and the white (you can take advantage of it for a salad).
2. Place a fine-mesh metal strainer over a bowl, tuck in the yolks, a few at a time, and mash them with a spoon.
3. Add the cold diced butter, icing sugar, a pinch of salt and mix with your fingertips.
4. Add grated lemon peel, flour, potato starch or cornstarch and quickly work all the ingredients until a homogeneous dough is left. You have to be quick so as not to overheat the dough.
5. Divide the dough into two parts, wrap them in plastic wrap and store in the refrigerator for at least 1 hour.
6. Prepare the baking sheet with parchment paper.
7. After resting, sprinkle the work surface with a little flour, remove one of the two doughs from the refrigerator and roll it out with a rolling pin until it reaches a thickness of 8-10 mm. If you have an adjustable rolling pin, it will be easier to make all the cookies the same. Don't take the second dough out of the fridge until you've finished with the first.
8. Use the cutter for canestrelli to remove the cookies, then with a smaller mold remove the

central hole. Keep putting the cookies on the tray as you prepare them.

9. Knead the leftover again to make more cookies. If the dough should be too sticky, wrap it again in transparent paper and store it in the freezer for a few minutes.

   Bake in a hot oven at 170° C for 12-15 minutes, until lightly browned.

   Let cool and sprinkle with icing sugar. They are kept for several days in a tightly closed jar.

Sicilian Cannoli, also with Thermomix

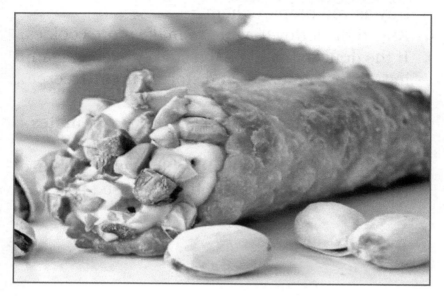

Servings 10

INGREDIENTS

- 125 g Wheat flour
- 30 ml Dry marsala or white wine
- Vinegar 1 teaspoon of coffee
- 20 g lard + 20 g spread
- 1 pinch salt
- 20 g icing sugar
- 20 g Egg yolk (1 egg approx, but weigh it)
- Lemon 1 just the skin
- Sunflower oil 1 liter
- 1 egg white
- For the filling
- 500 g Ricotta

- 120 g Icing sugar
- 30 g Chopped dark chocolate or chocolate drops
- To decorate
- Unsalted pistachios
- Chopped or dripped dark chocolate
- Candied fruit
-

PREPARATION

1. Put flour, sugar, salt, butter and the yolk in a bowl, mix with the tips of your fingers until you get a grainy dough. With thermo mix 20 sec speed 4.
2. Add wine, vinegar and the grated lemon rind. Knead first in the bowl and then transfer the dough on the counter until you get a smooth and homogeneous dough.
3. With Thermo mix 1,5 min spike or kneading mode.
4. Wrap it in plastic wrap and let it rest in the refrigerator for at least 30 minutes (you can also prepare it overnight).
5. After resting, divide the dough into 10 balls. Spread them very thin (about 2 mm) with a roller or with the pasta machine, giving it an oval shape.
6. Take a metal canutillo mold blank , spread it with a little lard. Place it on top of the dough and cut it into an oval shape about 10 cm. (The

first time you do it, I recommend you cut the dough so that it is a little shorter with respect to the length of the joint, about 8 cm, they will be smaller but this way it will be easier to extract it once fried). The dough that is left over in each cut, set it aside and knead it again to make more. Fold the dough on top of the joint first one side, brush the end with the whipped white, then close with the other half and press lightly so that the dough sticks in the place where you put the white.

7. Heat in a small pan but well wave abundant sunflower oil, it has to be enough so that the cannolo is well covered by the oil (not like mine). When it reaches 160-170° C (I put a citrus peel and when the oil is golden brown it will be ready). Dip a cannoli, fry it one by one by turning it over. If the dough has been very thin and the oil temperature is correct, the dough will fill with bubbles, turn the cannolo and remove it when it is well browned on all sides (it takes about 1 minute). Drain on kitchen paper. Let it cool slightly so that the joint is not too hot, then press it lightly to make it shrink and remove it from the cannolo.

8. I only have 3 metal joints so as soon as I cool the cannoli I remove them from the mold to make more.

9. Preparation of the cream

10. Put the ricotta to drain in a fine mesh strainer a few hours before (I the night before).

The next day throw away the serum, put the ricotta in a bowl and add the icing sugar, stir and add the chocolate. Stir again, put the cream in a pastry bag and reserve in the fridge.

11. Assembling the Sicilian cannoli
12. Prepare the bowls to decorate, one with pistachios, another with chocolate ...
13. Fill only the cannoli that you are going to eat and fill them just before eating.
14. Put the ricotta cream in a pastry bag and fill the joint so that the cream protrudes slightly.
15. Put the tip of the cannolo in the bowl with the chocolate shavings so that it sticks to the ricotta. Repeat on the other side.

Authentic Cantucci

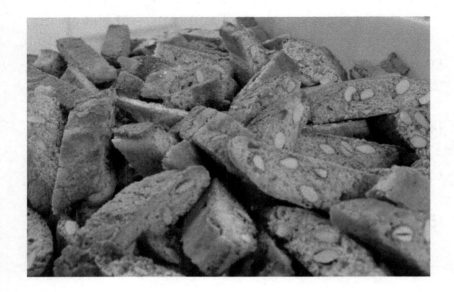

Servings 40

INGREDIENTS

- 350 g Flour
- 170 g Sugar
- 3 Eggs
- 100 g Butter at room temperature
- 10 g Yeast for desserts type Royal
- Vanilla essence a few drops
- 170 g Almonds with skin
- 1 Lemon or orange peel

To brush
- 1 Yolk

- 2 tablespoons milk

PREPARATION

1. Almonds are traditionally used with their skin on and raw. I prefer to toast them a little, I put them in the oven for about 20 minutes at 100° C. Let cool.
2. Put the 3 eggs, the grated citrus peel, the vanilla essence and the sugar in a bowl. Mix very well with a few rods until the sugar is almost dissolved.
3. Add flour and yeast, mix with a spatula and add creamy butter (it has to take time out of the fridge for it to be creamy). Knead with the spatula, or by hand if you prefer, until it is completely incorporated (the dough is sticky).
4. Add the almonds and knead to distribute them in the cookie dough.
5. Flour the countertop, pour the dough on top and divide it into 3 equal parts. With each one make a round churro about 4-5 cm wide. Place them on a parchment-lined cookie sheet.
6. Beat the yolk with 2 tablespoons of milk and brush the churros with it.
7. Bake in a hot oven at 180° C for 15-18 minutes. After the time has elapsed, remove from the oven, wait about 5 minutes so that they do not burn so much and cut the churros with a bread knife. You have to make oblique cuts, the cookies have to be 1.5-2 cm thick. Separate the

cookies between them and leave them standing (as in the photo). Bake another 5 minutes at 160° C. The authentic cantucci must be very dry. If you see that they are not ready yet, leave them in the oven for a while.

8. Once ready, let them cool before storing them in a tightly closed jar. They hold up very well for a month.

Chiacchiere

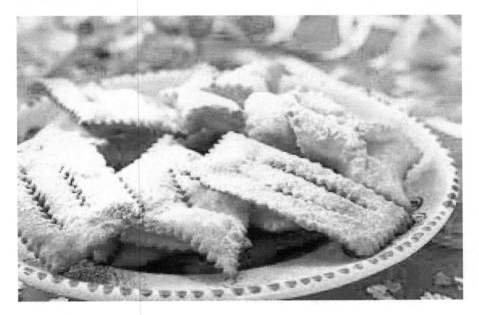

Servings 4

INGREDIENTS

- 300 g White flour
- 40 g Sugar
- 65 g Milk
- 30 g Soft butter
- Egg 1 large
- 2 tablespoons rum
- Orange or lemon streaked peel
- Sunflower oil for frying
- Powdered sugar for dusting

PREPARATION

1. Put all the ingredients in a bowl, mix and knead with your hands until they are all well amalgamated.
2. Wrap the dough in plastic wrap and let it rest for 20-30 minutes.
3. Cut small pieces of dough and roll it out very thinly with the help of a rolling pin or a pasta maker.
4. Then with the help of a short pasta wheel, cut the dough sheets into 2-3 cm wide strips
5. Put plenty of sunflower oil in a large skillet and put an orange or lemon peel inside. When the skin is golden, remove it and start frying the chiacchiere. Flip them over as soon as they start to inflate. Take them out as soon as they turn golden.
6. Drain on paper. Transfer them to a tray and as soon as they are cold, sprinkle them with plenty of icing sugar.

Coffee creamer glass

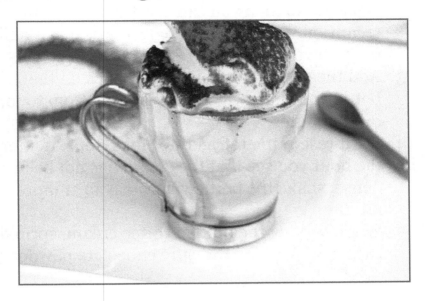

Servings 4

INGREDIENTS

- 70 ml Coffee (1 cup preferably from a coffee maker)
- 25 g Icing sugar
- 250 ml Whipping cream
- Pure cocoa powder to decorate

PREPARATION

1. Prepare the coffee in advance so that at the time of use it is very cold (if you put it in the refrigerator, better).

2. Put the icing sugar in a 1 liter bottle (better if it is plastic so then you can cut it to remove the cream) next to the coffee, cover and shake well to dissolve the sugar.
3. Add the cold cream, put the lid back on the bottle and shake vigorously from bottom to top for 5 minutes.
4. Let it rest in the refrigerator for 1 hour. If after the hour you see that the cream has not been dense, shake the bottle vigorously for 1 more minute.
5. When serving the bottled coffee cream, sprinkle each glass with a little pure chocolate powder.

cream bombs

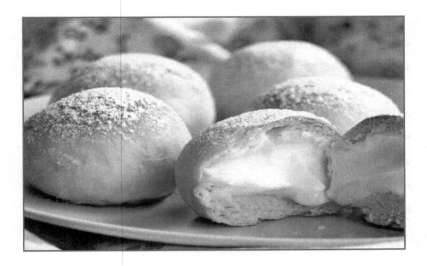

Servings 25

INGREDIENTS

- 170 g W360 strength flour from El amasadero
- 170 g Common wheat flour
- 200 ml Whole milk
- 55 g Sugar
- 10 g Fresh baker's yeast
- 30 g Butter at room temperature
- 1 Vanilla bean

For the cream
- 200 g Ricotta
- 200 g Whipping cream
- 35 g Glass sugar

- Organic half lemon peel

For the heavy cream
- 270 ml Milk
- 80 g Sugar
- 15 g Honey
- 25 g Cornstarch
- 1 Vanilla bean
- To sprinkle
- Cb Icing sugar
-

PREPARATION

1. Heat the milk to 37° and dissolve the yeast in it first, then the sugar. Open the vanilla pod and put the seeds in the milk.
2. Put the two flours in a bowl, add the warm milk. Mix first with a spoon, then knead with your hands. Transfer the dough onto your work surface and knead for about 5 minutes.
3. Cut the butter into pieces, roll out the dough and place a piece in the center. Knead until the butter is completely absorbed, then add another piece of butter and knead again. Keep going until all the butter is gone.
4. Put the dough in a bowl previously greased with oil or butter, cover with plastic wrap and let it rest in a warm place for 2 hours. While preparing the heavy cream.
5. After resting, divide the dough into portions of 30 g each. Fold each portion on itself as I show

you in this video and then roll the dough. Traslada el bollito is a baking tray covered with greaseproof paper. When you finish, cover the buns with plastic wrap and let it rest in a warm place for 1 hour and a half. While you finish preparing the creams.

6. Brush the buns by mixing a yolk with about 50 ml of milk. Bake the buns in a hot oven for 12-15 minutes at 160°. It is very important that they are tender and not toasted.

7. Preparation of the buns with Thermomix

8. Put milk, yeast, sugar and the seeds of a vanilla bean in the glass. Program 1.5 min 37° speed 2.

9. Add the flours for 3 min in the spike or kneading mode.

10.   Divide the butter into small portions. Operate the machine in herringbone or kneading mode and add the butter little by little while the machine is running. Do not add the next piece of butter if the first has not been absorbed.

11. Continue with step 4 of the traditional method.

12. Milk cream

13. Put milk, sugar and the seeds of the vanilla bean in a saucepan. Dissolve the sugar over medium heat.

14. Add the honey and dissolve it helping you with some rods.

15. Add cornstarch and cook over medium heat for a few minutes until it thickens without stopping stirring with the rods.

16. With Thermomix: Put milk, sugar, honey and the vanilla bean seeds in the glass for 2 min 37° speed 3. Add cornstarch 4 min 90° speed 3.
17. Ricotta cream

Put the ricotta with the icing sugar and the zest of half a lemon in a bowl. Mix until you get a uniform texture.

In another bowl, whip the cream to firm snow. Then add the ricotta and mix gently with a spatula from bottom to top.

Assembling the fiocchi di neve

Stir the heavy cream vigorously with a stick to remove the lumps that form when stirring after it has cooled. Add the heavy cream to the cream cheese and stir gently from bottom to top with a spatula. Put the cream in a piping bag with a long, narrow nozzle.

When filling the buns it is important that they are still TEMPERED, in this way the crumb will give way to make room for the cream.

Fill the buns with the cream by pinching them on the side or at the base. Enter the cream slowly, you will see how the bun will puff up.

Let cool and sprinkle with icing sugar. At my house they don't usually arrive the next day so I leave them at room temperature covered with cling film or under a hood.

Chocolate and hazelnut

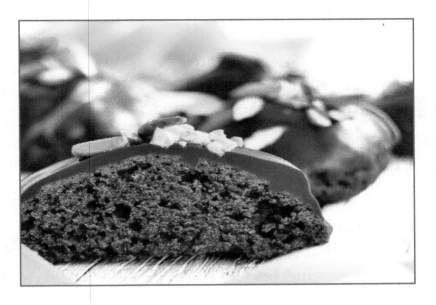

Serving: 35

INGREDIENTS

For the cookies
- 400 g Flour
- 170 g Sugar
- 240 ml Milk
- 75 g Pure chocolate powder
- 120 g Butter (at room temperature)
- 2 tablespoons orange marmalade
- 1 tablespoon honey
- Ground cinnamon a pinch
- Orange 1 (skin only)
- Yeast for desserts (Royal type) 1 sachet

- Cloves 4
- 1 pinch salt
- For coverage
- 200 g Dark chocolate
- 35 g Butter
- Unsalted pistachios for garnish
-

PREPARATION

1. Heat the milk in a glass and melt the honey inside.
2. Scratch the orange peel and crush the cloves with a mortar and pestle. Put them in a bowl with all the ingredients (the butter has to be at room temperature), add the milk. Mix first with a spatula and then knead a little by hand until you get a homogeneous dough.
3. Moisten your palms, scoop up a walnut-sized piece of dough, shape it into a round or oval shape, then flatten it. Place the cookies on a parchment-lined cookie sheet.
4. Bake in a hot oven at 180° C for 16-18 minutes. When the chocolate and orange cookies are ready, transfer them on a rack and let them cool completely.
5. Melt the chocolate together with the butter and mix well. Try not to exceed 40-50°C so it will be shiny.
6. Take a cookie by the ends of the base and dip only the top of the cookie in the chocolate.

Reheat the chocolate a little as needed. Sprinkle with pistachios at the end of each cookie and leave them on the rack until the chocolate hardens. Store the chocolate and orange cookies in a tightly closed container or under a glass bell.

Cookies

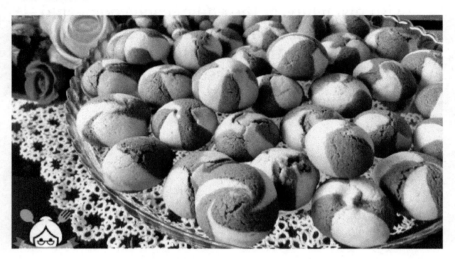

Servings 25

INGREDIENTS

- 200 g Wheat flour
- 30 g Maizena (corn starch)
- 90 g Powdered sugar
- 80 g Butter
- 8 g Yeast for desserts
- 50 g Cream for desserts (whipping 35% fat)
- 1 Vanilla bean
- Egg 1 small (40 g)

PREPARATION

1. Put flour, cornstarch, icing sugar and yeast in a bowl and stir to mix all the ingredients well.
2. Add the butter cut into pieces and mix with the tips of your fingers until you get a grainy mixture.
3. Add the cream and the seeds of the vanilla bean. Knead a little with your hands.
4. Beat the egg and add it to the batter. Knead a few seconds in the bowl and then transfer the dough on the counter. Work it just a little bit, until you get a smooth and uniform dough. Wrap in plastic wrap and let it rest in the refrigerator for at least 30 minutes.
5. After resting, sprinkle the countertop with a little flour and roll the dough out to about 8 mm thick. Cut the cookies with a cutter (the traditional way is the one in the photograph) and carefully transfer them to a cookie sheet lined with greaseproof paper.
6. Bake in a hot oven at 180° C for 15 minutes. Once ready, wait until they are warm to move them. When they are cold, store them in a glass jar or tin box.

Fifteen jelly

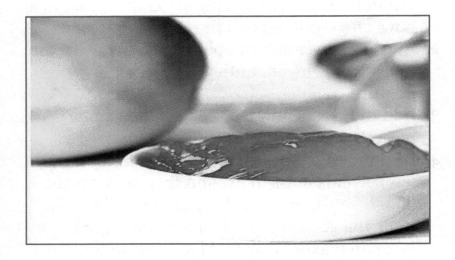

Servings 4

INGREDIENTS

For the gelatin
- 2 kg Quinces
- 2 L Water
- 2 Lemons
- 350 g Sugar
- 9 g Agar

For the fifteen jam
- 750 g Cooked quinces
- Lemon 1
- 5 g Ginger
- 300 g Sugar

PREPARATION

1. Wash the quinces well and cut them into pieces of the same size, removing the seeds.
2. Put the fruits in a pot together with the lemon juice and the water that has to cover the fruits (I 2 liters). Cook first over high heat and when it starts to boil lower the heat, cook until the fifteen are tender (about an hour and a half).
3. Put a fine cloth or gauze in a colander, place it over a pot and pour the quinces on top, let it drain well for a few hours.
4. Place the pot with the filtered liquid (mine was 1.2 liters) on the fire, when it starts to boil add the sugar and stir until it dissolves.
5. Dissolve the agar with a little cold water and pour it into the boiling liquid. Cook for another 3 minutes.
6. Pour the quince jelly into previously boiled glass jars. If you want to keep the gelatin for a long time, put the jars tightly closed in a bain-marie and let it boil for 20 minutes.
7. For the jam or quince paste
8. I have divided the quinces into two batches. Grind the quinces with a robot, put them in a pot together with the sugar and lemon juice or cook over low heat, stirring often until they reach the desired consistency (10 minutes for jam, 15-20 for fifteen paste).
9. Pour the quince jam into previously boiled glass jars. If you want to keep it for a long time, put

the jars tightly closed in a bain-marie and let it boil for 20 minutes.

Strawberry ice

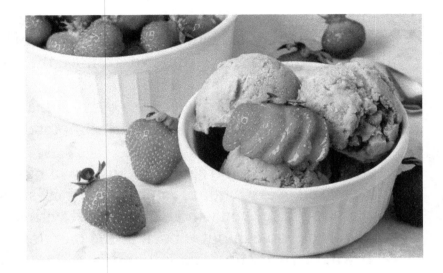

Servings 4

INGREDIENTS

- 600 g Clean strawberries
- 120 g White sugar (or white sugar 90 and 30 g invert sugar)
- Juice of half a lemon
- 200 ml Water

PREPARATION

1. Put a saucepan with the water and sugar on the fire and boil for 2 minutes. When ready let cool completely.

2. Meanwhile, put the strawberries in a bowl and add the lemon juice. With a mixer, beat at maximum power until a very fine puree has been left (the time will depend on the mixer).
3. Pass through a fine strainer to remove the seeds (optional).
4. Mix the strawberries with the cold syrup and mix again with the blender until completely mixed.
5. Put in a taper and freeze. The slush will have to be mixed every 2 hours to prevent ice crystals from forming. You can go crushing it with a spoon or you can put it back in the blender.
6. It will be ready in 15-24 hours depending on the freezer.
7. To make it irresistible, take it out of the freezer half an hour before serving and mash with a spoon to make it creamier. Serve with whipped cream on top or accompanied by a delicious Sicilian brioche.
8. Preparation with Thermomix
9. Put the water with the sugar in the glass and program 4 minutes, 100°, vel. 2. When ready, pour the syrup into a bowl to cool completely.
10. Wait a few minutes for the glass to return to normal temperature, then without rinsing it put the clean strawberries and lemon juice inside, we program 20 seconds, vel. 8.
11. When the syrup is cold, add it to the strawberry puree and program 10 seconds vel. 8.
12. Pour everything into a taper and freeze.

13. Every 2 hours we will pass the granita through our Thermomix at vel. 7 and helping us at the same time with the spatula until the slush achieves a uniform texture. We will repeat this step 3 times.
14. To make it irresistible and even creamier, take it out of the freezer half an hour before serving and crush it with a spoon or go over it in the Thermomix at high speed. 7 helping you with the spatula. Serve with whipped cream on top or with a delicious Sicilian brioche.

Stracciatella ice cream

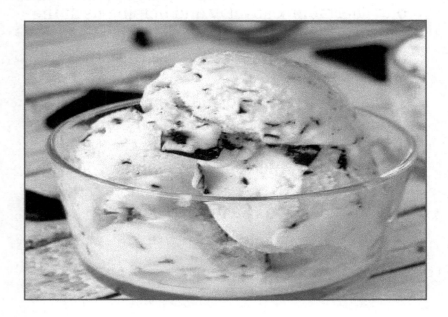

Servings :4

INGREDIENTS

- 90 g White sugar
- 20 g 35 g or 30 g Dextrose of invert sugar
- Skimmed milk powder
- 4 g Locust bean gum
- 400 g Whole milk
- 120 g Asturian cream for desserts 30% fat
- 60 g Dark chocolate

PREPARATION

1. Put in a bowl sugar, dextrose (if you use invert sugar add it in step 3), powdered milk and locust bean gum, mix everything very well.
2. Put milk and cream in a saucepan, heat over medium-low heat until reaching 40° C, stirring all the time.
3. Add the contents of the bowl that you have prepared before (if you use invert sugar add it now) and stir until it reaches 80° C (try not to exceed them), once the temperature is reached, stir another couple of minutes. When you finish, pour everything into a tapper and let it rest in the refrigerator for at least 6 hours.
4. Put in a bowl sugar, dextrose (if you use invert sugar add it in step 3), powdered milk and locust bean gum, mix everything very well.
5. Put milk and cream in the glass, program 2.5 minutes 50° C vel. two.
6. Add the content of the bowl that you have prepared before (if you use invert sugar add it now) and program 5 minutes 80° C vel. 2.5. When you finish, pour everything into a tapper and let it rest in the refrigerator for at least 6 hours.
7. Ice cream preparation
8. Prepare the refrigerator, without placing the ice cream basket. Take the ice cream mix out of the refrigerator and mix very well with a whisk. When you have it ready, take the ice cream

basket out of the freezer, place it in the refrigerator and turn it on so that the butterfly begins to rotate. Pour the preparation into the refrigerator little by little from the opening and butter for approximately 40 minutes.

9. While you put in the freezer the container where you will put the ice cream and melt the dark chocolate in a double boiler or in the microwave. Spread the chocolate on greaseproof paper and put it in the fridge or freezer. Let stand 10 minutes. Take out the chocolate sheet and by folding the sheet, remove the chocolate from it, without handling it too much so that it does not melt again. Store in the freezer

   for a couple of minutes, take it out again and just break the chocolate into a ball with the paper. Add the laminated chocolate to the ice cream about 5 minutes before turning off the refrigerator.

   When the ice cream is ready (it will take approximately 35-40 minutes and it will have occupied the entire basket), transfer it to a very cold container, store it in the freezer for 1 hour before serving.

Hazelnut coffee

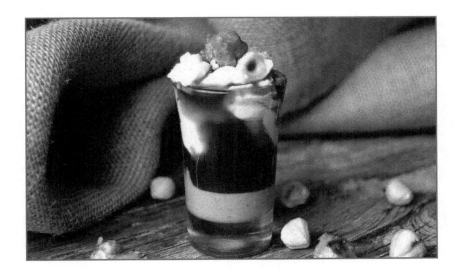

Servings 4

INGREDIENT

For the caramelised hazelnuts
- 40 g roasted hazelnuts
- 30 g White sugar
- 1 tablespoon water
- For the hazelnut cream
- 100 g Hazelnuts
- 1 tablespoon icing sugar
- For the final presentation
- Espresso 4
- 100 ml Whipping cream
- 1 teaspoon sugar

PREPARATION

1. Caramelised hazelnuts
2. Put a non-stick frying pan on a very strong fire with the sugar and water and without mixing.
3. When the sugar begins to melt, lower the heat and add the hazelnuts. Mix with a wooden spoon until the hazelnuts are sugar-coated and dark, about 8 minutes.
4. As soon as they are ready, pass them on parchment paper until they are completely cold.
5. You can prepare it and have it ready for when you need it by storing it in a tightly closed glass jar
6. Hazelnut cream
7. Grind the hazelnuts with a robot, until you see that they transform into a smooth and shiny cream.
8. Add a tablespoon of icing sugar and continue crushing until you get a uniform consistency.
9. You can keep it in a tightly closed glass jar.
10. Preparation of coffee with hazelnuts
11. Prepare the coffees.
12. Whip the cold cream with a tablespoon of sugar.
13. Put two tablespoons of the hazelnut spread in the bottom of the glass.
14. Add the sweetened coffee to your liking up to the middle of the glass.
15. Put the whipped cream on top of the coffee and garnish with the caramelised hazelnuts.

16.Serve hot

Migliaccio, Also with Thermomix

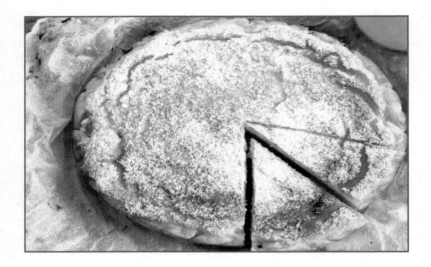

Servings 5

INGREDIENTS

- 800 ml Whole milk
- 1 vanilla bean (or essence)
- 50 g Butter
- Orange 2
- Lemon 1
- 200 g Durum wheat semolina from El Amasadero
- 300 g Ricotta
- Eggs 4
- 250Sugar
- Salt a pinch
- A 22-24 cm mold

PREPARATION

1. Put milk, 50 g of sugar, the seeds of a vanilla bean, the skin of an orange and a lemon without the white part in a saucepan. Cook over medium heat until it comes to a boil, stirring occasionally. Remove the skins from citrus fruits.

2. Add the semolina in the rain little by little while stirring with a few rods. There must be a thick cream that peels off the walls. Remove from the heat, add the butter and stir until it is completely melted and incorporated. Once ready, transfer it to a large plate and cover with transparent film. Let cool completely.

3. In a bowl put the eggs, the grated skin of an orange, a pinch of salt and the remaining sugar (200 g). Beat with an electric stirrer until you get a voluminous and clear mixture (takes about 7-8 minutes).

4. Add the ricotta and continue mixing with the rods until fully incorporated.

5. When the semolina cream is completely cold, add it little by little to the eggs mounted with the ricotta and beat with the rods until no lumps remain.

6. Spread a 22-24 cm mold with butter and then flour it or place a previously wet and drained greaseproof paper. Pour in the migliaccio mass and smooth the surface with a spatula.

7. Bake in a hot oven at 180° C for 50-60 minutes. It has to be golden on top. To see if it is ready, do the stick test, you will notice the cake very soft but the stick will come out clean.
8. Wait until it is cold to unmold.
9. It is a cake that is even richer the day after it is made. You can keep it out of the fridge for a maximum of a couple of days, or in the fridge for a longer time. I assure you that cold is even richer.

Coffee mousse

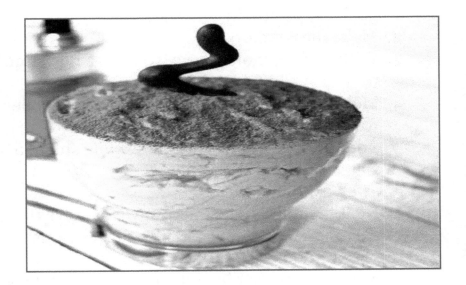

Servings 6

INGREDIENTS

For the mousse
- Ristretto or espresso coffee cup
- 150 ml Whipping cream 35% mg
- 150 g White chocolate
- Buds 2
- 50 g Milk
- 3 g Gelatin in sheets or two sheets
- For the glasses
- 200 g Dark chocolate
- 6 plastic cups
-

PREPARATION

1. Soak the gelatin in cold water.
2. Make the coffee.
3. With a whip, mount 2 egg yolks in a bowl until they turn whitish and foamy.
4. Melt the chopped chocolate in a double boiler with the coffee cup.
5. Add the yolks to the chocolate while still in a water bath and stir well with the whip. Get away from the fire.
6. Heat the milk in the microwave, dissolve the gelatin in it and now add it to the previous preparation.
7. Now pour everything into a bowl and let it cool. Stir well every little bit. When it is very cold, mount the cream and add it little by little with enveloping movements from the bottom up. You can whisk again with the whips if there are lumps of cream. Store in the fridge for a couple of hours.
8. To prepare the chocolate glasses, chop the chocolate and melt it in the microwave or in a bain-marie, heat it to the minimum necessary and start pouring it into the glasses until the entire surface is completely covered. Make sure that the entire edge of the glass is very thick. Store them in the fridge as soon as you finish them but take them out a few minutes before so they don't break when you unmold them. Fill the glasses helping you with a pastry bag.

Cherry mousse, also with thermomix

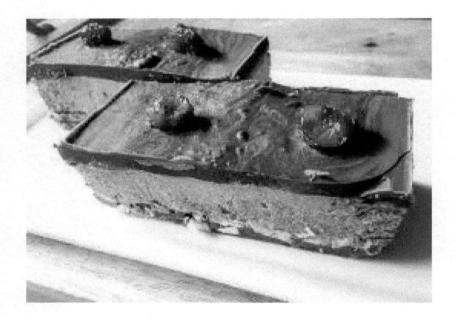

Servings 6

INGREDIENTS

- 650 g Pitted cherries (1kg whole cherries)
- 3 L Egg whites
- 300 ml Cream 35% fat
- Cream of tartar the tip of a teaspoon (or a few drops of lemon juice)
- Juice of half a lemon
- 200 g Sugar
- 5 Gelatin sheets

PREPARATION

1. Put a bowl to whip the cream in the fridge.
2. Wash the cherries and remove the pit.
3. Pn in a saucepan with the juice of half a lemon and 150 g of sugar and cook over medium heat for 25 minutes.
4. When this time has elapsed, mash the "jam" as well as possible with the help of a robot. Then pass it through a strainer. Set aside a glass of "jam" that we will use to coat the mousse.
5. Soak the gelatin sheets.
6. When the "jam" is warm, around 50° C, add the well-drained gelatin sheets and mix well until they are completely dissolved.
7. While the jam is cooling completely, mount the whites. As soon as they start to froth add 50 g of sugar and beat until they are fully assembled, that would be until when, if you turn the bowl over, the whites remain stuck and do not fall.
8. Once the jam is cold you can whip the cream.
9. Join the "jam" with the cream, little by little and making enveloping movements. When the mixture is homogeneous, add the whites mounted little by little and always with enveloping movements so that the mousse does not lose its air.

10.   Distribute the cherry mousse in a few glasses or jars and cover the surface of each one with the "jam" that you had set aside.
11. Let cool for about 4 hours and that's it.
12. Elaboration with thermomix
13. Put the pitted cherries, the lemon juice and 150 g of sugar in the glass. Program 25 minutes, 100° C temperature and speed 2.
14. When it is ready program 1 minute speed 10. We reserve a glass of "jam", it will serve to cover the mousse.
15. When the temperature of the jam reaches 60°C, add the previously hydrated gelatin sheets and mix for 30 seconds on speed 4. Reserve the "jam" in a bowl and let it cool completely.
16. Wash the glass well, dry it perfectly.
17. Place the butterfly in the glass and mount the whites together with a pinch of cream of tartar for 3 minutes speed 3.5. Add the sugar that is left in the middle of the process. Reserve in a bowl.
Wash the glass and the butterfly well, dry them and put them in the freezer for 10 minutes.
When the vastus is very cold, whip the cream with the butterfly at speed 3.5. Do not program the time and watch by looking when the stripes begin to form. It will take 1 to 2 minutes for them to appear.
Put the cream in a bowl add the "jam" little by little making enveloping movements. When the mixture is completely homogeneous, add the

whites mounted little by little and always with enveloping movements so that our mousse does not lose air.

To make a cake

The steps to follow are the same, you will only have to add two more gelatin sheets.

You also have to prepare a base of 150 g Maria type cookies with 70 g of butter.

You can use a 22 cm diameter mold.

CONCLUSION

The Mediterranean diet is based on the eating habits of the southern countries. Foods rich in vitamins, minerals and fiber such as fruit, vegetables, legumes and low-fat dairy products such as sheep or goat milk are the main nutritional components of the Mediterranean diet.

Almonds, herbs, whole grain products and garlic are also on the daily menu. Food such as red meat, which is often very fatty, as well as fatty dairy products such as cream cheese or cream quark should be avoided in the Mediterranean diet.

However, if you look closely, the Mediterranean Diet is more of a way of eating and living than a diet. You can only lose weight in connection with sport. The number of calories, which is not taken into account in the Mediterranean diet, should also be taken into account. The nutritional principle attaches importance to a healthy lifestyle, which is characterized by a cozy, slow and enjoyable celebration of food.

Lightning Source UK Ltd.
Milton Keynes UK
UKHW021256100521
383453UK00001B/108